CONCISE GUIDE TO

Psychopharmacology and Electroconvulsive Therapy

American Psychiatric Press

CONCISE GUIDES

Robert E. Hales, M.D.
Series Editor

CONCISE GUIDE TO

Psychopharmacology and Electroconvulsive Therapy

Laurence B. Guttmacher, M.D.
Associate Professor of Psychiatry
Director, Somatic Therapies Service
Director, Residency Education
Department of Psychiatry
University of Rochester
School of Medicine and Dentistry
Rochester, New York

American Psychiatric Press, Inc.

Washington, DC
London, England

American Psychiatric Press, Inc.
1400 K Street, N.W., Washington, DC   20005

Library of Congress Cataloging-in-Publication Data
Guttmacher, Laurence B., 1947–
    Concise guide to psychopharmacology and electroconvulsive therapy
    /Laurence B. Guttmacher. —
        p.   cm. — (Concise guides / American Psychiatric Press)
    Rev. ed. of: Concise guide to somatic therapies in psychiatry.
    © 1988.
    Includes bibliographical references and index.
    ISBN 0-88048-340-7 (alk. paper)
    1. Mental illness—Chemotherapy—Handbooks, manuals, etc.
2. Psychopharmacology—Handbooks, manuals, etc.
3. Electroconvulsive therapy—Handbooks, manuals, etc.
I. Guttmacher, Laurence B., 1947–   Concise guide to somatic
therapies in psychiatry. II. Title. III. Title: Psychopharmacology
and electroconvulsive therapy. IV. Series: Concise guides (American
Psychiatric Press)
    [DNLM: 1. Mental Disorders—therapy—handbooks. 2.
Psychotropic Drugs—therapeutic use—handbooks. 3.
Electroconvulsive Therapy—
methods—handbooks.   WM 39 G985c 1994]
RC483.G88   1994
616.89′18—dc20
DNLM/DLC
for Library of Congress   93-5676
                                                                CIP

British Library Cataloguing in Publication Data
A CIP record is available from the British Library.

This book is for Terry, Joshua, and Rachel, who showed remarkable tolerance and love during the very strange hours that this work demanded.

CONTENTS

INTRODUCTION

to the *American Psychiatric Press Concise Guides*

The American Psychiatric Press Concise Guides series provides, in a most accessible format, practical information for psychiatrists—and especially for psychiatry residents and medical students—working in such varied treatment settings as inpatient psychiatry services, outpatient clinics, consultation/liaison services, and private practice. The Concise Guides are meant to complement the more detailed information to be found in lengthier psychiatry texts.

The Concise Guides address topics of greatest concern to psychiatrists in clinical practice. The books in this series contain a detailed table of contents, along with an index, tables, and charts, for easy access; and their size, designed to fit into a lab coat pocket, makes them a convenient source of information. The number of references has been limited to those most relevant to the material presented.

The selection and proper use of psychopharmacological agents and electroconvulsive therapy is an important clinical concern that every practitioner must face. Laurence B. Guttmacher, M.D., has a wealth of academic and clinical experience in educating residents about their use. He begins this *Concise Guide to Psychopharmacology and Electroconvulsive Therapy* by presenting an approach to pharmacological decision making and by highlighting 19 rules that psychiatrists should consider in their general approach to medication usage. Dr. Guttmacher also summarizes some basic pharmacological principles pertinent to psychoactive medications. This Concise Guide emphasizes those somatic treatments used to treat the most common disorders: antipsychotics, antidepressants, lithium, carbamazepine, electroconvulsive therapy, and anxiolytics.

Of particular interest to psychiatrists are the effects of aging on a medication's pharmacokinetics. Dr. Guttmacher includes a chapter on geriatric psychopharmacology that summarizes the use of psychotropic medications in this population and informs physicians about the management of agitation and dementia. He also includes a chapter on the psychopharmacological treatment of other psychiatric disorders of special clinical significance: aggression, alcoholism, cocaine abuse, eating disorders, panic disorders, and others.

This book is organized to provide the physician with basic and applied information needed to make treatment decisions. The *Concise Guide to Psychopharmacology and Electroconvulsive Therapy* is an accessible, easy-to-use reference that can be readily available when making pharmacological recommendations. Dr. Guttmacher has written an outstanding, compact, and portable guide.

Robert E. Hales, M.D.
Series Editor
American Psychiatric Press Concise Guides

PREFACE

The 5 years since the first edition, *Concise Guide to Somatic Therapies in Psychiatry,* serve as vivid testimony to just how short the half-life is for knowledge in this field. Clozapine, which represents a fundamentally different approach to schizophrenia, reached the market in 1991 accompanied by considerable controversy about how to manage its attendant toxicity and how to make it financially accessible to those in need. Fluoxetine withstood largely unfounded charges that it somehow induced suicidality. Other serotonin-specific, reuptake-inhibiting antidepressants are now arriving. Bupropion, another antidepressant with a different mechanism of action, returned to the market. Valproate emerged as an alternative to lithium or carbamazepine in the treatment of bipolar disorder. New work with atypical depression has led to a better understanding of the potential of monoamine oxidase inhibitors. There is a better appreciation of the risks of thymoleptics in pregnancy.

The list could go on for a long time. These refinements in our approach must be tempered with the realization that, with the possible exception of clozapine, there have been no fundamental breakthroughs. It is impossible to anticipate what the next edition of this book will bring, but it seems clear that psychopharmacology will remain a wonderfully exciting aspect of the field.

With appreciation for my residents
and students, who make this area so exciting
for me, and for my patients,
who make it so important.

INTRODUCTION

This book provides an overview of psychopharmacology. It is intended for those who are beginning to work in the area and for others who might be seeking a quick refresher. These pages contain many facts. However, if this book succeeds, it will convey something more important: it will teach the reader how to think like a psychopharmacologist. This skill is transferable to other branches of medicine and nonpharmacological therapeutics as well. The logic and approach should be the same whether the clinician is choosing an antipsychotic, determining which antibiotic to use for pneumonia, or even deciding whether to institute family or individual psychotherapy.

■ APPROACHES TO PHARMACOLOGICAL DECISION MAKING

Document those signs and symptoms that are amenable to pharmacotherapy and are useful indicators of the patient's overall clinical state.

Clinicians should document in writing the signs and symptoms they are targeting before instituting treatment. Failure to do this is a common clinical error. If this is not done, the physician may be confronted several weeks later with a completely new set of problems and will not be sure if the difficulties are iatrogenic or are part of the original illness. Start by picking several target behaviors and assess the severity of the problems before writing the first prescription. The simple approach is, for example, to target early morning awakening, anorexia, diurnal variation, and suicidal ideation and rate them at 70, 80, 65, and 55, respectively, with 100 representing the maximal possible intensity. Alternatively, standard rating scales such as the Hamilton Depression Scale or the Brief Psychiatric Rating Scale could be used serially to monitor progress (1, 2).

Establish a meaningful set of differential diagnoses.

A patient can present to the emergency room with exactly the same findings from ingesting cocaine, experiencing schizophrenia, or having meningitis. Haloperidol might help the resultant behavior with all three, but it would probably be unnecessary for the patient who ingested cocaine because the psychosis is likely to resolve on its own. In the case of meningitis, haloperidol would certainly be a less desirable treatment than penicillin. Primary psychiatric differentials are greatly facilitated using structured diagnostic interviews like the Structured Clinical Interview for DSM-III-R (3). At a minimum, the *Diagnostic and Statistical Manual of Mental Disorders,* Fourth Edition (DSM-IV) (4), should be routinely consulted.

Obtain a detailed drug history.

If a patient has responded to imipramine during two previous episodes, there is no reason to begin nortriptyline. If a patient previously has been dystonic when challenged with haloperidol, the clinician should use another antipsychotic or should prophylactically administer an anticholinergic. It is important to obtain family histories of response or toxicity to particular agents, especially if there is no better way to decide among various agents.

Do not begin drug treatment before completing steps one through three. The only exception should be for frank emergencies, and these are decidedly rare.

There is almost always time to stop and think. This requires the ability to resist internal pressure, as well as pressure from nursing staff, to jump in and do "something." Remember that "doing something" without a well-thought-out rationale may lead to complications and serious consequences.

If a patient is taking clinically significant doses of medication that are not causing toxicity when first encountered, continue the medication while you are performing your initial evaluation.

Failure to attend to this principle leads to confusion between withdrawal effects and undertreated primary illness.

Whenever possible, avoid changing more than one variable at a time.

This rule is generally honored in the breach because it is rarely possible to isolate variables this cleanly; we frequently take patients away from work, admit them, begin family and activities therapy, and start an antipsychotic simultaneously. Much of this cannot and should not be avoided, but it is almost always possible to avoid more than one pharmacological manipulation at a time. If a tricyclic and an anticholinergic are simultaneously added and the patient gets either better or worse, it will be impossible to determine which was responsible. Always try to avoid simultaneously tapering off one medicine and beginning another.

Within a group of drugs, you must prescribe on the basis of side effects; no convincing data exist to support differences in efficacy.

There are no data to indicate that one antipsychotic is any better than another if used in comparable doses; the same can be said for anxiolytics and antidepressants. They differ in terms of their toxicity. One patient's toxicity may be another's good outcome. Sedation may be a desired side effect for one patient and a problem for another. Toxicity, then, is the basis for choosing a particular drug. At times a judgment must be made about whether the possibility of orthostasis and sedation would be worse for the patient than the possibility of extrapyramidal symptoms.

Establishing a dose is done by titrating benefit versus toxicity.

Unfortunately, long-delayed toxicities such as tardive dyskinesia must be entered into the cost-benefit equation. Dosage changes should reflect the patient's overall clinical state, not just day-to-day fluctuations. There are few absolute ceilings on doses.

Psychotropics treat symptoms, not diseases.

Antidepressants treat early morning awakening, diminished libido, and anorexia—not depression. Likewise, until we really understand the pathogenesis of schizophrenia, we will have to be content with treating hallucinations and delusions with antipsychotics, while being relatively ineffective at addressing the amotivation and impaired judgment that are as much a part of the illness as the more "positive" symptoms.

Avoid medications that can obscure the collection of valuable data.

One would never prescribe an antipyretic to a patient with pneumonia at the start of antibiotic treatment. The same sort of reasoning dictates that hypnotics not be prescribed for patients with insomnia secondary to a primary psychiatric disorder—sleep is simply too valuable an indicator of a patient's clinical state, and insomnia almost invariably corrects itself several days before the depression lifts or the mania clears. Because of this, the presence or absence of insomnia is an important guide about whether the patient is taking the right drug or the right amount of the medication.

Enlist your patients in a collegial fashion in fighting their illness.

The physician needs to enlist patient cooperation. The idea should be that although the clinician knows about psychopharmacology, the patients know what they are experiencing. Success is far more likely if problems are approached jointly.

Compliance is one of the most difficult problems in psychopharmacology (5, 6).

The quality of the doctor-patient relationship is the single strongest predictor of compliance. The chance of compliance will be enhanced by exploration of your patients' attitudes toward medications before prescribing them. It is vital that you educate your patients and their families. They must understand the treatment plan before it is begun. Failing to explain that imipramine will take several weeks to work invites the patient to discontinue it, because the side effects will long antedate the therapeutic response. Estimates of noncompliance in psychiatry vary widely, but it seems probable that one-fifth of schizophrenic inpatients and one-half or more of schizophrenic outpatients do not take their medication as prescribed. There are some ominous predictors of noncompliance—ego-syntonic grandiose delusions, social isolation, and past history of defaulting with medication—that should lead to special efforts to enhance compliance. Complex medication regimens, with multiple medications and times of administration, increase the likelihood of noncompliance. Side effects and high cost of medications also contribute significantly to noncompliance.

The ideal patient is one who is motivated to give up his or her symptoms, is on only one affordable drug that is taken once a day, experiences few side effects, and is willing to engage actively in treatment. The ideal physician is willing to devote considerable energy and time toward forging a relationship with the patient and his or her family, is able to hear feedback from them, is willing to educate them about the medicine, and is able to see medication as part of a larger treatment program.

Consider cost when prescribing.

One antidepressant may cost 20 or 30 times more than another. There may be special indications for an expensive drug's use, but there are few reasons to routinely use such a compound as a first-line agent. The patents for many psychotropics are now expiring, so generic alternatives are becoming available. The tables in each chapter include an indication of which drugs are available generically. There are few convincing data to suggest significant differences in bioequivalence among various preparations used in psychiatry, with the exception of medications for children. If a stable patient's condition deteriorates, every effort should be made to learn whether a new generic drug was used, but such instances are rare.

Table 1–1 lists the cost to the pharmacist for some psychotropics. The cost to the patient will be higher after the pharmacy adds its markup. Prices will vary significantly for a drug after its patent protection ends and competition develops from generic preparations.

TABLE 1–1. **Drug wholesale prices for pharmacists**

Drug	Typical daily dose (mg)	Cost to pharmacist ($)
Antipsychotics		
Chlorpromazine	300	.10
Clozapine[a]	100	3.42
Fluphenazine decanoate	25[b]	7.60
Fluphenazine HCl	5	.63
Haloperidol	5	.04
Haloperidol decanoate	50[c]	27.94
Loxapine	25	.76
Mesoridazine	100	.81
Molindone	25	.78
Thioridazine	200	.19
Thiothixene	5	.18
Trifluoperazine	10	.11
Anticholinergics		
Benztropine	4	.08
Diphenhydramine	25	.02
Antidepressants		
Amitriptyline	200	.07
Amoxapine	150	.42
Bupropion	300	2.08
Clomipramine	150	2.47
Desipramine	200	.57
Doxepin	200	.25
Fluoxetine	20	2.01
Imipramine	200	.13
Maprotiline	200	1.24
Nortriptyline	100	2.63
Paroxetine	20	1.75
Phenelzine	60	1.40
Sertraline	100	1.63
Tranylcypromine	30	1.16
Trazodone	300	.38
Thymoleptics		
Carbamazepine	600	.31
Divalproex	1,000	1.63
Lithium carbonate	900	.13

Note.   Prices are average wholesale price to the pharmacist. Where generic products are available, the cheapest preparation was chosen.
[a]The usual cost for clozapine and requisite monitoring is near $5,000 annually. [b]Normally a 2-week supply. [c]Normally a 3- to 4-week supply.
Source.   From *Annual Pharmacists' Reference, 1993 Red Book*. Montvale, NJ, Medical Economics, 1993.

Avoid polypharmacy.

There is never any reason to give more than one drug from a particular class. There are, however, times when more than one class of drugs needs to be prescribed. Toxicity is often additive within a drug class, but desirable effects are not. For instance, all conventional antipsychotics act by blocking the dopamine receptor, but they differ from one another in respect to the other receptors they affect. These other receptors cause much of the toxicity. Adding a second antipsychotic will only lead to unnecessary toxicity, which could be avoided simply by increasing one drug to a more appropriate level of dopamine blockade. This will become clearer when we discuss mechanisms of action in each chapter.

Never use a fixed-combination drug.

Fixed-combination drugs are allegedly constructed to enhance patient compliance. In fact, they may do the opposite. Generally, the constituents are present in such small doses that many pills would have to be taken to achieve the desired effect. Moreover, the prices of fixed-combination drugs are high. Most important, there is great loss in terms of flexibility; one cannot raise and lower the combined medications independently. A psychotic depression may require an antipsychotic and an antidepressant initially, but the antipsychotic should be lowered as the psychosis clears, whereas the antidepressant should be maintained. Such a manipulation would be impossible with a fixed-combination drug.

Dealing with an acute episode is different from prophylaxis.

Electroconvulsive therapy (ECT) is the most effective treatment for an acute episode of depression, yet it has little demonstrated efficacy for the prevention of relapse. Lithium is effective for the prevention of recurrent unipolar depression but has relatively little to offer as an acute antidepressant.

Don't try to learn about all the psychotropics.

There are simply too many of them. Pick a smaller group and become comfortable with them. Thorough knowledge of four antipsychotics, three antidepressants, two benzodiazepines, one anticholinergic, and lithium should suffice for almost all patients.

Maintain a healthy skepticism of new products and prescription trends.
Jeste and Wyatt coined the term "Law of the New Drug" when they pooled the studies of deanol, a cholinergic agonist, in the treatment of tardive dyskinesia (7). In the first year, 100% of studies reported positive results; after that, there was a steady decline until the fifth year, when all studies reported negative results. You should expect to be assaulted by advertising for every new drug, but beware of this.

There are no rules.
All rules are based on populations of patients. Individual patients may well be outliers. The population of manic patients probably require lithium levels of 0.8–1.5 mmol/L for acute treatment, but individual patients may be best treated with levels of 0.3 or 2.0 mmol/L.

■ LEGAL ISSUES

Many of the treatments suggested in this book go beyond indications approved by the United States Food and Drug Administration (FDA). Use of imipramine in panic disorder patients and carbamazepine in bipolar patients are well-accepted therapies within the psychiatric community, but these indications are not specifically approved by the FDA. It is perfectly appropriate and defensible to use such treatments because they are well within community standards (8). It is important, however, to document your rationale for doing so. The most effective actions to prevent litigation are forming a good relationship with your patient, obtaining meaningful informed consent, documenting carefully what you have done, and behaving responsibly.

Unless otherwise noted, doses suggested are for average-sized, medically intact adults. No mention will be made of children or adolescents, and geriatric patients will be addressed in a separate chapter.

■ BASIC PHARMACOLOGY

Kinetics

The *effective amount of a drug* reflects a dynamic equilibrium among absorption, distribution, metabolism, excretion, and, for psychiatry, the ability to cross the blood-brain barrier. Understanding these concepts will allow individualization of drug regimens to reflect changes with the aging process, drug interactions, or many physical impairments.

Gastric absorption is increased on an empty stomach, because direct mucosal contact is possible. Most psychoactive drugs are weak bases and are therefore best absorbed at the higher pH of the jejunum. Empty stomachs accelerate gastric emptying, which leads to more rapid contact with the area where most absorption occurs. The net result is that empty stomachs are associated with rapid onset of action. Rapid onset is not always desirable. Some drugs are embedded in a relatively nonabsorbable material in an attempt to slow absorption and provide a more gradual, smoother onset. Most drugs diffuse into the body. This process is facilitated by small, nonionized, lipid-soluble molecules. Note that these are the same factors that are predictive of lipophilicity and of crossing the blood-brain barrier. It therefore follows that most psychoactive compounds are rapidly absorbed.

The *volume of distribution* is a theoretical construct defined as the amount of the drug in the body divided by the amount of the drug in plasma. Very lipophilic drugs, which is to say most psychoactive compounds, have large volumes of distribution. This is associated with a long half-life.

The *distribution phase* is the dispersion of the drug into tissue. Only free, unbound drugs will cross cell membranes. Psychotropics are highly bound to plasma proteins, notably albumin and glycoprotein. Only a small percentage of the drug is therefore available to the site of action, the brain.

The *blood-brain barrier* is not a specifiable place, but rather a functional system. Many drugs can be at high concentration peripherally and low level in the brain, or vice versa. This distinction is accounted for by the blood-brain barrier. Even though blood flow in the brain is remarkably high, drugs are slow to penetrate because brain capillaries lack the fenestrations seen peripherally and brain parenchyma is tightly packed, with little extracellular fluid.

With the notable exception of lithium, most psychotropics are metabolized hepatically. In some instances, the drug's effects are dependent on this because only the metabolites are psychoactive. In other cases, metabolism may be a part of clearing the drug from the body. Metabolism may also be complicated by a number of factors. The first-pass effect can be of major importance; 90% of fluphenazine HCl is metabolized before reaching the systemic circulation. This is why so many intramuscular preparations are more potent on a milligram-per-milligram basis than their oral congeners. Some drugs may stimulate hepatic enzymes responsible for their own degradation or that of other drugs. Patients on benzodiazepines will require more barbiturate before ECT. Carbamazepine induces hepatic enzymes in a predictable fashion, so that levels dip after 3–5 weeks on the drug.

A drug's clearance reflects how it is removed from the body—this is one of the determinants of a drug's half-life. There are multiple half-lives, and imprecision often obscures which is being described. The *plasma half-life* is a measure of how long it takes to remove half of a drug from plasma, is the easiest to measure, and is therefore most commonly used. The *biological half-life* is the time necessary to remove half of a drug from the body. The *pharmacological half-life* is the time necessary to halve a drug's pharmacological effect. It is important to realize that drugs with long half-lives will take a long time to reach steady state and a long time to be cleared. Steady state is reached in about four to five half-lives. Dosage intervals less than two-thirds the half-life will be associated with minimal fluctuation in level once steady state is reached.

The Neuron and Sites of Action

Figure 1–1 represents a pair of idealized neurons. A neurotransmitter is synthesized in the presynaptic neuron, transported down the axon, and stored in presynaptic vesicles that can be extravasated, dumping the transmitter into the synaptic cleft. Here the transmitter can latch onto receptors, which can be either presynaptic or postsynaptic. The presynaptic receptors are typically autoreceptors that regulate further synthesis and the release of more transmitter. The postsynaptic receptors will effect some response, frequently through the use of a second messenger. The effects of the transmitter will end in one of three ways: enzymatic degradation, diffusion, or reuptake into the presynaptic cell.

There are two determinants of receptor occupancy: *1)* the

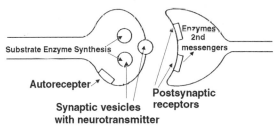

FIGURE 1–1. **The neuron and sites of action.**

affinity of the receptor for the ligand and 2) the amount of the ligand in relation to the number of receptors. Receptors are in a state of dynamic equilibrium. The rate of synthesis for most is fixed, but the rate of degradation varies widely. Typical half-lives are in the range of 10–100 hours.

Ligands may be agonists or antagonists. Agonists effect a biological response. Partial agonists have weak biological activity and compete for binding, but produce less of a response than a full agonist. Noncompetitive antagonists fully occupy receptors but produce no response. Binding is irreversible and no agonist will bind, no matter how high the concentration. The effect is to shift the drug-response curve to the right, also depressing the maximum possible response. Competitive antagonists, by contrast, can be overcome by sufficiently high concentrations of an agonist. In that

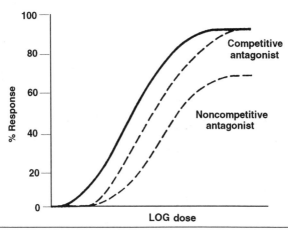

FIGURE 1–2. **Drug response curves for competitive and noncompetitive antagonists.**

situation the curve is shifted to the right (Figure 1–2). The ED_{50} is that dose of a drug that will effect half the maximal drug response.

Denervation hypersensitivity occurs after prolonged occupation of a receptor by an antagonist. More receptors are created and there is an increase in the avidity of the receptor for the ligand. This increase in receptor number and affinity is referred to as *upregulation*. The opposite situation—a decrease in the number of receptors and affinity for the ligand—is referred to as *downregulation*.

■ REFERENCES

1. Williams JBW: A structured interview guide for the Hamilton Depression Rating Scale. Arch Gen Psychiatry 45:742–747, 1988
2. Overall JE, Gorham DR: The Brief Psychiatric Rating Scale. Psychol Rep 10:799–812, 1962
3. Spitzer RL, Williams JBW, Gibbon M, et al: User's Guide for the Structured Clinical Interview for DSM-III-R. Washington, DC, American Psychiatric Press, 1990
4. American Psychiatric Association: Diagnostic and Statistical Manual of Mental Disorders, 4th Edition. Washington, DC, American Psychiatric Association, 1994
5. Blackwell B: Treatment adherence. Br J Psychiatry 129:513–531, 1976
6. Chen A: Noncompliance in community psychiatry: a review of clinical interventions. Hosp Community Psychiatry 42:282–287, 1991
7. Jeste D, Wyatt RJ: Therapeutic strategies against tardive dyskinesia. Arch Gen Psychiatry 39:803–816, 1982
8. Apler WD: "Off-label" uses of approved drugs: limits on physicians' prescribing behavior. J Clin Psychopharmacol 9:368–370, 1989

■ ANNOTATED GENERAL REFERENCES

American Medical Association: AMA Drug Evaluations. Chicago, IL, American Medical Association, 1993
   A three-volume set that is updated quarterly covering all of pharmacology.

American Psychiatric Association: Benzodiazepine Dependence, Toxicity, and Abuse: A Task Force Report of the American Psychiatric Association. Washington, DC, American Psychiatric Association, 1990
   A very well thought-out discussion of this topic.

American Psychiatric Association: The Practice of Electroconvulsive Therapy: Recommendations for Treatment, Training, and Privileging: A Task Force Report of the American Psychiatric Association. Washington, DC, American Psychiatric Association, 1990
   Another very well thought-out discussion.

Ciraulo DA, Shader RI, Greenblatt DJ, et al (eds): Drug Interactions in Psychiatry. Baltimore, MD, Williams & Wilkins, 1989
   A complete, spiral-bound reference.

Cooper JR, Bloom FE, Roth RH: The Biochemical Basis of Neuropharmacology. New York, Oxford University Press, 1991
   An amazingly well-written review of basic transmitter and receptor work.

Gelenberg AJ, Bassuk EL, Schoonover SC: The Practitioner's Guide to Psychoactive Drugs. New York, Plenum, 1991
   A good basic, spiral-bound psychopharmacology reference.

Goodwin FK, Jamison KR: Manic Depressive Illness. New York, Oxford University Press, 1990
   A superb reference on everything relating to bipolar disorder.

Guy W: ECDEU Assessment Manual for Psychopharmacology.

Washington, DC, US Department of Health, Education and Welfare, 1976
  A wonderful compendium of rating scales.

Jefferson JW, Greist JH, Ackerman DL, et al: Lithium Encyclopedia for Clinical Practice, 2nd Edition. Washington, DC, American Psychiatric Press, 1987
  A masterful compendium of all matters relating to lithium.

Meltzer HY (ed): Psychopharmacology: The Third Generation of Progress. New York, Raven, 1987
  Multiple authored and therefore erratic, but still an excellent library reference.

Rizack MA, Hillman CDM: The Medical Letter Handbook of Adverse Drug Interactions. New Rochelle, NY, The Medical Letter, 1989
  A wonderful place to look for troublesome interactions.

Salzman C: Clinical Geriatric Psychopharmacology. New York, McGraw-Hill, 1992
  A brief book that superbly covers the field.

ANTIPSYCHOTICS

■ **HISTORY**

Chlorpromazine was synthesized in 1950. Two years later, Delay and Deniker began to work with it in France. Its effects were so obvious that they knew they had an effective treatment for psychosis after they had treated their first 10 patients. In 1955 chlorpromazine began to be used in the United States. Largely as a result of its introduction, the state hospital population dropped dramatically. The decreased census is accounted for by a dramatic reduction in the average length of stay, not a drop in the number of admissions. Although some of this may be attributed to the community mental health center movement of the 1960s and the recent resurgent interest in deinstitutionalization, antipsychotics have been the most important factor in emptying the state hospitals.

During the four decades of experience with these drugs there have been cycles in prescribing practices. We have vacillated between high-dose, aggressive treatment and more moderate courses of medication. Increasing awareness of the effects of serious toxicity, such as tardive dyskinesia and neuroleptic malignant syndrome, has recently led to a movement back to more temperate use. See Table 2–1 for a list of important antipsychotics.

The most recent addition to the antipsychotic pharmacopoeia is clozapine. This is a drug with a significantly different mechanism of action. It is accompanied by a different side-effect profile and has a real chance of benefiting some of the most treatment-refractory schizophrenic patients. Because of its unique qualities, clozapine is discussed in a separate section beginning on page 45. All other discussion of antipsychotics should be presumed to refer to conventional dopamine D_2 receptor antagonists.

TABLE 2–1. Important antipsychotics

Generic name (by class)	Trade name	Dose equivalent (mg)	Comments
Phenothiazines			
Aliphatic			
chlorpromazine[a]	Thorazine	100	The original antipsychotic, the prototypic low-potency agent.
Piperidine			
thioridazine[a]	Mellaril	95	The only antipsychotic with an absolute maximum, 800 mg/day, because of pigmentary retinopathy at higher doses. Very anticholinergic.
mesoridazine	Serentil	50	A first-pass metabolite of thioridazine.
Piperazine			
trifluoperazine[a]	Stelazine	5	An early phenothiazine.
fluphenazine[a]	Prolixin	2	Also available as fluphenazine decanoate and enanthate. These are depot forms for which dose equivalents are not available.
	Permitil		
Dibenzoxazepine			
loxapine[a]	Loxitane	15	
Dihydroindolone			
molindone	Lidone	10	Possibly associated with weight reduction.
	Moban		

Thioxanthenes[a] thiothixene[a]	Navane	3	Has a very high incidence of akathisia.
Butyrophenone haloperidol[a]	Haldol	1.6	The prototypic high-potency drug. A decanoate form is available. Dose equivalents for it are not available.
Dibenzodiazepine clozapine	Clozaril	50	Has minimal effects on the D_2 receptor, leading to questions about mechanism of action. Minimal extrapyramidal syndromes. High affinity for α_2-adrenergic, muscarinic, and H_1 receptors. Very sedating. Agranulocytosis requires weekly blood counts.
Diphenylbutylpiperidines pimozide	Orap	2	Approved only for Tourette's disorder.

[a] Available generically.

■ MECHANISM OF ACTION

Clozapine represents the first real breakthrough in the pharmacology of this area since the introduction of chlorpromazine. With its possible exception, all antipsychotics appear to act by blocking the postsynaptic dopamine receptor. Dopamine-depleting agents, such as rauwolfia alkaloids (e.g., reserpine), also have antipsychotic efficacy, but toxicity limits their use. Otherwise, progress has been limited to the development of longer-acting depot drugs designed to enhance compliance and agents of varying potency with slightly differing toxicities.

Standard antipsychotics can be seen as occupying a continuum from high to low potency. This is another way of saying that it takes more milligrams of chlorpromazine than of haloperidol to have the same effect. Table 2–1 includes a column for equivalent doses that can be used as a guide for ordering the drugs this way. Low-potency drugs, such as chlorpromazine, are more sedating, cause more orthostasis, are more likely to have anticholinergic effects, and probably are associated with greater lowering of the seizure threshold than high-potency agents, which are more likely to be associated with extrapyramidal syndromes and neuroleptic malignant syndrome.

Because all antipsychotics act by blocking the D_2 receptor, it follows that they all have similar efficacy if given in equivalent doses. Antipsychotics block other receptors as well. Some of the other effects are listed in Table 2–2. The varying effects on histamine H_1, α-adrenergic, and muscarinic receptors go a long way toward predicting toxicity.

Understanding these principles makes it clear why *two antipsychotics should never be coprescribed*. Toxicity is additive, but the desired effect—blockade of the D_2 receptor—is no greater when two drugs are used than it would be when higher doses of one compound are taken.

■ INDICATIONS

Antipsychotics, like other psychotropics, treat symptoms, not diseases. These drugs are highly effective in treating target symptoms such as agitation, assaultiveness, hallucinations, delusions, and psychomotor excitement arising from a wide variety of etiologies. They are not, however, antischizophrenic or antimanic per se. The following is a discussion of some of the leading indications grouped by diagnostic category. Even though they are listed by diagnosis, it should be remembered that these drugs treat signs and symptoms, not diagnoses.

TABLE 2-2. **Receptor affinities of antipsychotics**

Drug	D_2 affinity	Standardized H_1 affinity	Standardized α_1 affinity	Standarized muscarinic affinity
Chlorpromazine	1	1	3	2
Thioridazine	1	1	3	3
Mesoridazine	1	3	3	2
Loxapine	1	3	2	2
Molindone	0/1	0/1	0/1	2
Trifluoperazine	2	0/1	0/1	0/1
Fluphenazine	4	0/1	0/1	0/1
Thiothixene	4	0/1	0/1	0/1
Haloperidol	3	0/1	1	0/1
Clozapine	0/1	4	4	4

Note.   Data are based on in vitro receptor binding assays with human brain tissue. Standardized affinity = affinity for the given receptor ÷ D_2 affinity. 0 = no effect; 4 = marked effect.
Source.   Adapted from Black JL, Richelson E: "Antipsychotic Drugs: Prediction of Side-Effect Profiles Based on Neuroreceptor Data Derived From Human Brain Tissue." *Mayo Clinic Proceedings* 62:369–372, 1987.

Schizophrenia, Schizophreniform Disorder, and Brief Reactive Psychoses

The overwhelming majority of antipsychotics are prescribed for patients with schizophrenia. Review of the target symptoms mentioned above indicates that the medications are quite effective in treating the positive symptoms of schizophrenia but are relatively ineffective at addressing the important negative symptoms of the disorder, such as impaired judgment and insight, amotivation, and flattened affect. These target symptoms do respond at times, albeit slowly, so it is generally worth attempting to address these issues pharmacologically, though they often are most responsive to social skills training and supportive and educational psychotherapy.

Acute Phase

Several years ago there was enthusiasm for very aggressive initial treatment of thought disorders. This was variously termed *psychotolysis, psychiatric digitalization,* or *rapid neuroleptization.* Psychotic patients were given haloperidol 5–10 mg im every 30–60 minutes until their psychosis cleared. This approach was remarkably well tolerated, but we subsequently learned that the outcome measured a week or more later was no better than that of more moderate treatment. There is still room for this sort of treatment, but it should be reserved for the truly dangerous patient who poses a substantial risk of harm to self or others. This sort of aggressive use of pharmacotherapy is probably most appropriately termed *rapid tranquilization,* for it assists behavioral control acutely but will probably not treat the underlying delusions, hallucinations, or conceptual disorganization in the long term (1).

Rapid tranquilization involves a relatively simple technique; haloperidol 5 mg im can be given initially, followed by 10 mg po every 30 minutes until behavioral control (usually sedation) is realized. If patients reject the oral form, then 5 mg im can be substituted. It is highly unusual for more than three doses to be required; no more than five should be given. Although the initial dose of this regimen is parenteral, subsequent doses should be offered orally. The rationale is that parenteral administration is slightly more rapid in onset, but the difference is not great enough to require continuous intramuscular use. In cases in which an even more rapidly acting agent is required, droperidol 5–10 mg can be used. Droperidol is a butyrophenone, closely related to haloperidol, that is used as an anesthetic agent because of its very rapid onset. It is only available in parenteral form. No more than three doses should be given. All of these approaches should be regarded as similar to the management of alcohol withdrawal or diabetic ketoacidosis; treatment is keyed around continuous evaluation. There can be no absolute guidelines about dosing; it should be a matter of frequent reevaluation and titration.

Recently, in an attempt to minimize antipsychotic exposure, there has been interest in combining neuroleptics with benzodiazepines (BZDs). Lorazepam 1–2 mg im is most frequently used because it is the only BZD with dependable parenteral absorption. Acute use of parenteral BZDs seems to offer comparable results to those obtained with parenteral antipsychotics (2). Combinations of BZDs and antipsychotics may lead to a somewhat more rapid response than either alone, but any advantage is lost after the first week (3).

In the usual nonemergent situation, use a slower, more thoughtful approach. The first steps should involve obtaining a good patient history and thinking about differential diagnosis. The cornerstones of this method of thinking are outlined in Chapter 1. Once the history is obtained, the diagnosis reasonably defined, baseline unmedicated behaviors noted, and realistic target behaviors plotted, initial pharmacotherapy can be attempted. Use of a standardized rating instrument such as the Brief Psychiatric Rating Scale (4) at baseline and weekly thereafter is a useful, reproducible way to document the impact of treatment.

Initial Nonacute Management

The goal now switches from behavioral control to treatment of more fundamental defects. The aim of pharmacotherapy should be the treatment of hallucinations, delusions, sleep alterations, mannerisms, stereotypies, and disorders of communication. Negative symptoms such as lack of motivation, difficulty initiating activities, and diminished insight, judgment, and affect respond more rarely, but are legitimate behaviors to attempt to treat nonetheless.

Selection of the appropriate antipsychotic should depend on which toxicities the particular patient will tolerate best. A recently catatonic patient should not ordinarily receive a high-potency agent for fear of inducing a dystonia that might be misinterpreted. Another patient who had concerns about his masculinity would do better with a high-potency agent because it would minimize the chance of erectile dysfunction. Remember to pay attention to whatever did or did not work pharmacologically with previous episodes. Past experience is always the best predictor of response.

Selection of an initial dose should depend on size, level of agitation, degree of psychosis, smoking status, and other relevant factors. Normative initial daily doses are approximately 5 mg of haloperidol, 200–300 mg of chlorpromazine, or the equivalent dose of another antipsychotic agent. The dose can be increased every 3–5 days, but the practitioner must realize that it may take as long as 6 weeks for an antipsychotic to take effect. There are no data to establish that doses much beyond 15 mg/day of haloperidol offer any increased benefit (5). Doses as low as 20 mg/day of haloperidol will often be associated with subtle toxicity including akinesia and amotivation as early as the second week of treatment (6). For several of the high-potency drugs there is a strong suggestion that there is a *therapeutic window* or a curvilinear dose-response curve (7). With this type of drug, a dose that is too high is every bit as ineffective as one that is too low. The difficult part of this phase of treatment is resisting the pressure to move too quickly. The urgency will come from the physician, the patient, the patient's family, and concerned staff, all of whom will sense the patient's pain and want immediate intervention to end it. Unfortunately, there seems to be a specific time frame that cannot be accelerated. Overly vigorous initial treatment may expose the patient to drugs that are not necessary and may even retard progress. Patients who smoke clear antipsychotics more rapidly and will require significantly higher doses (8).

The Treatment-Refractory Patient

Patients refractory to conventional treatment during the initial phase pose a special challenge. When patients fail to respond to 6 weeks of a moderate dose of an antipsychotic, a series of questions should be asked:

1. Is the patient correctly diagnosed? Failure to respond to conventional treatment should always lead to diagnostic doubt. The possibilities are many but could include a major depression with psychotic features, drug toxicity, endocrine disorders, substance abuse, or a primary neurological disorder.

2. Is the patient in fact taking the medication? It is difficult to overestimate the extent of noncompliance.

3. Is the patient absorbing the drug appropriately? Antipsychotic plasma level measurements are available from many commercial laboratories. Given the enormous variability in plasma levels for any given dose, there is considerable theoretical appeal for their use. They should, however, at this stage be interpreted with considerable caution. Their use makes most sense for patients who have failed to respond to usual doses or where there is confusion about toxicity. For several antipsychotics there is a suggestion of a curvilinear dose-response curve. Whether very high doses are associated with diminished response or increased toxicity is often difficult to know. Akathisia, for example, is often subtle and difficult to discern from the agitation of worsening psychosis. It is clear, however, that some patients who have been treatment refractory may improve with lowering of their dose. There is especially strong support for this approach with high-potency agents. Decisions such as these may be facilitated by antipsychotic level measurements (9).

Tentative guidelines are shown in Table 2–3 for "therapeutic" plasma levels for some antipsychotics. Although laboratories will report on many agents, the data are either unavailable or contradictory for antipsychotics other than those listed. If a patient is doing well, then any levels different from those should either be ignored or, preferably, never elicited. The other reason for considering antipsychotic levels is when there is concern about drug interactions. Carbamazepine, the most common example, may induce hepatic microenzymes and lead to diminished antipsychotic levels. Antipsychotic levels should be drawn once steady state is achieved and 12 hours after the last dose for oral medications.

One does, on occasion, see patients who respond to depot, injectable antipsychotics but not to oral agents. It is not clear whether this represents a form of malabsorption, enhanced compliance, or some other phenomenon, but use of a parenteral agent can provide a legitimate alternative for the patient who has not responded to an oral medication. The possibility that a patient is an outlier who requires higher than normal doses of medication should always be seriously considered before switching to another compound. In the absence of toxicity an increase of dose should be one of the first steps in treating the refractory patient.

TABLE 2–3. **Antipsychotic plasma levels**

Drug	Tentative therapeutic plasma level (ng/ml)
Chlorpromazine	30–100
Fluphenazine	0.2–2.0
Haloperidol	2–12
Perphenazine	0.8–2.4

Source. Data from Van Putten T, Marder S, Wirshing WC, et al: "Neuroleptic Plasma Levels." *Schizophrenia Bulletin* 17:197–216, 1991.

4. Is the patient unresponsive to one antipsychotic but a candidate for another? The clinician rarely sees patients who fail to respond to one compound but respond quite well to another. Usually it is wisest to switch to a completely new class of drugs (e.g., from a phenothiazine to a butyrophenone or a dihydroindolone).

If a patient has failed to respond to several antipsychotics, including oral and parenteral forms, then there are other possibilities to be considered (10). The best-supported alternative is clearly clozapine, which is discussed later in this chapter. Benzodiazepines, lithium, or carbamazepine may be used to augment the effects of antipsychotics. These are discussed in Chapters 4 and 6.

Electroconvulsive therapy is an alternative to drug therapy that can help some schizophrenic patients (see Chapter 5). Megadoses of antipsychotics have never been shown to be of benefit in controlled trials, but individual patients clearly have benefited, and daily doses as high as 1,200 mg of fluphenazine HCl seem remarkably well tolerated (11).

Nonbiological treatments should not be overlooked. Behavioral and family treatments can be quite effective. Insight-oriented techniques should probably still be viewed as experimental with this population, but can be of significant benefit to certain individuals (12).

There are no scientific data to support the use of megavitamins, β-blockers, dialysis, or psychosurgery. Each has had its vogue, but has passed from the scene. The danger of such approaches is that they hold out a false promise to patients and their families.

Maintenance Treatment

In maintenance treatment the aims are to maintain the gains of the initial phase, perhaps even furthering them, and to prevent the return of acute illness. Once again, biological treatment should be integrated into a broader program including psychological, occupational, and family interventions.

How long to maintain a patient on pharmacotherapy is the art, rather than the science, of psychopharmacology. Frequent, severe prior episodes that occurred without much of a prodrome would be persuasive arguments for more prolonged maintenance. The presence of insight into the developing illness is vital if a patient's medication is to be safely discontinued. A strong family history of schizophrenia and poor premorbid functioning increase the likelihood that medicine will need to be maintained. The quality of the clinician's relationship with the patient and his or her family is a very important part of the decision making. A trusting relationship will give you access to the data needed to assess:

1. How likely the patient is to deteriorate
2. How much warning there will be
3. How difficult a decompensation would be to bring under control
4. How likely the patient would be to seek help

When maintenance neuroleptics are discontinued, they should be tapered slowly. Antipsychotics are highly lipophilic drugs that, as a result, take a long time to be cleared from the body. It is not unusual for a patient to decompensate several months after stopping medication. Typically, the patient fails to make an association between the suspension of the medicine and the psychotic break; compliance is therefore not fostered. This long latency between discontinuing medication and the resulting decompensation should encourage a very slow, gradual tapering of the medication over the course of several months. There are three possible outcomes:

1. Decompensation may occur rapidly, indicating the need for resumption of the full dose of medication.

2. Breakthrough of some symptoms may occur, indicating that an intermediate dose should be maintained.
3. The patient may do very well, indicating that no medicine is necessary.

Maintenance with antipsychotics should probably be reserved for schizophrenic patients; the risk of tardive dyskinesia is higher for patients with affective disorders, and there are few other indications for prolonged treatment (13).

It is clear that lowering the dose leads to diminished toxicity. It is equally evident that very low doses lead to a greater likelihood of relapse (14). This leaves the clinician in a real dilemma, which is further complicated by the often substantial delay before the full impact of a diminished dose is evident.

Mania

Both lithium and carbamazepine work well in acute treatment for mania. Antipsychotics simply make the response somewhat more rapid. If used, they should be for the short term only, with prophylaxis offered by one of the thymoleptics. The possibility of substituting benzodiazepines for some or all of a neuroleptic regimen during an acute manic episode is being explored, but is not yet well supported.

Psychotic Depression

The ranking of efficacy is

1. Electroconvulsive therapy
2. A combination of an antipsychotic and an antidepressant
3. An antidepressant alone
4. An antipsychotic alone (15)

Once again, it should be emphasized that patients generally should not be maintained on antipsychotics because antidepressants usually will do an effective job without exposing patients to the risk of tardive dyskinesia.

Dementia and Delirium

Antipsychotics have long been used to treat agitation in patients with dementia. They will, at times, be helpful, but it should be realized that treatment is largely empirical. The few good, controlled trials available suggest that high-potency agents are preferred and that, as with schizophrenia, they are helpful with agitation, assaultiveness, hyperactivity, and hallucinations, but not with apathy or withdrawal (16). The significant anticholinergic impact of low-potency antipsychotics in cognitively compromised patients means that high-potency agents should be used except with patients who are already parkinsonian. The initial dose should be approximately one-third to one-fifth of that used with younger patients. An adequate trial should last at least 1 month. In delirium, brief use of an antipsychotic may be helpful in obtaining behavioral control while the primary cause is addressed. A similar strategy to that described in the section on acute management earlier in this chapter is appropriate.

Anxiety

Antipsychotics are reasonably efficacious anxiolytics, but they should not be used as such given their toxicity and the availability of alternative agents and approaches.

Tourette's Disorder

Haloperidol 0.5–5 mg/day is helpful for both the motor and vocal tics of Tourette's disorder. Pimozide has been approved by the Food and Drug Administration only for the treatment of this disorder. Doses usually range from 0.5 to 9 mg/day (17). Higher doses have been associated with bradycardia and Q-T interval prolongation on electrocardiogram, so this drug should probably be reserved for patients who are either unresponsive to haloperidol or experiencing problems with it. Clonidine has also been of benefit and may have less potential toxicity. Hypotension often limits how much can be given, and the desired effects of the drug may not be seen for several months. Typical doses may range from 0.15 to 0.60 mg/day.

■ SIDE EFFECTS

Common, Early Side Effects

Because of their blockade of the dopamine receptor, antipsychotics can cause signs and symptoms that so closely mimic idiopathic parkinsonism as to be indistinguishable from it. These extrapyramidal syndromes (EPS), which include dystonias, parkinsonism, and akathisia, are more likely to occur with high-potency antipsychotics, may wax and wane, will disappear with sleep, and may increase with emotional stress. The likelihood of a drug inducing EPS correlates highly with its ability to block the dopamine receptor.

Acute dystonias classically occur within 1–5 days of the initiation of treatment or with an increase in dose. Common presentations include opisthotonos, torticollis, and oculogyric crises, but almost any part of the body can be involved. Rarely, laryngeal involvement can occur, at times being so severe as to require intubation. Dystonias are most common with young males. These reactions are extremely frightening to an unprepared patient, so all young male patients, especially outpatients, should be forewarned about this possibility and encouraged to seek prompt treatment. Treatment is with diphenhydramine 25–50 mg or benztropine 1–2 mg iv. Patients will respond within minutes.

Drug-induced parkinsonism presents with all of the signs associated with idiopathic Parkinson's disease, including masked facies, cogwheeling, three-cycle-per-second tremor, festinating gait, stiffness, and drooling. Peak risk appears between 5 and 75 days after initiating treatment or after increasing the dose. Routine use of a standardized examination to monitor EPS is encouraged. A slightly modified version of a commonly used examination is included in Table 2–4. The treatment of EPS is to decrease the dose, to switch to a lower-potency drug, or to treat with one of the agents listed in Table 2–5. If one of these drugs is used, it should be reviewed within several weeks to months, because they generally can be withdrawn. All too often antiparkinsonian drugs are routinely maintained, exposing patients to needless expense and toxicity.

All of the antiparkinsonian drugs listed have short half-lives and should be prescribed on a two or three times daily basis. The half-lives of antipsychotics are much longer. Anticholinergics and related compounds therefore should be continued for several days after the discontinuation of an antipsychotic. Anticholinergics are not without toxicity. The mnemonic about atropine can be extended to other anticholinergics and should be remembered: "dry as a bone, red as a beet, blind as a bat, mad as a hatter." Constipation, visual blurring, erectile dysfunction, and urinary retention, especially in patients with enlarged prostates, should be added to the litany of potential problems associated with anticholinergic effects. Amantadine differs because it is a dopamine agonist. It is significantly more expensive, and there is a question about whether its effectiveness is maintained over the long term, but it does provide an alternative to anticholinergic toxicity in vulnerable patients. It should also be remembered that low-potency agents, especially thioridazine, mesoridazine, and clozapine, are potent anticholinergics in their own right. Combination of these drugs with other anticholinergic agents, including many tricyclic antidepressants such as amitriptyline, can leave a patient vulnerable to delirium.

Akathisia differs from other forms of EPS. It is a purely sensory phenomenon, typically presenting as a poorly described sense of restlessness, usually felt most strongly in the legs, that causes people to pace. Patients may have difficulty remaining seated throughout an interview and will frequently shift about, crossing and uncrossing their legs. Unlike other forms of EPS, tolerance rarely develops to this symptom. The period of maximal risk is from 5 to 60 days after exposure. Frequently this is misdiag-

---

TABLE 2–4. **Suggested examination for extrapyramidal syndromes**

---

1. Observe gait, paying particular attention to arm swing, and posture.

   0 = normal; 1 = decreased arm swing; 2 = No. 1 plus obvious rigidity; 3 = stiff gait, arms rigid before abdomen; 4 = stooped, shuffling with propulsion and retropulsion.

2. You and the patient should stand with arms extended to the side at shoulder height. On a signal let them drop.

   0 = normal with loud slap and rebound as they hit the side of the body; 1 = slowed drop, little rebound; 2 = no rebound; 3 = markedly slowed, no slap; 4 = arms fall very slowly as if against resistance.

3. Rotate elbow and monitor the wrist with your other hand. Rate both arms separately for stiffness and cogwheeling. The same procedures can be done for the legs. Rate on a 0–4 basis.

4. Have patient hold out hands. Observe tremor then and at rest.

   0 = normal; 1 = mild finger tremor; 2 = tremor of finger and hands; 3 = limb tremor; 4 = whole body tremor.

5. Have patient open his or her mouth and raise his or her tongue to assess salivation.

   0 = normal; 1 = pooling with maneuvers above; 2 = occasional problems with speech because of drooling; 3 = as with 2, but frequent; 4 = frank drooling.

6. You and the patient should place your hands on a table. Begin to tap your index finger as rapidly as possible. Repeat with both hands. Monitor for bradykinesia.

   0 = normal; 1 = mild slowing; 2 = moderate slowing; 3 = severe slowing; 4 = virtually immobilized.

Source. Adapted from Simpson GM, Angus JWJ: "A Rating Scale for Extrapyramidal Side Effects." *Acta Psychiatrica Scandinavica* 212 (suppl):11–19, 1970.

nosed as agitation, leading to an increase in the antipsychotic, when what is needed is a decrease, a switch to a lower-potency agent, or treatment with an anticholinergic or a β-blocker. Compared with the other forms of EPS, akathisia is the least likely to respond to antiparkinsonian drugs. A trial may well be warranted nonetheless. Alternatively, treatment with propranolol 20–60 mg/day, or the equivalent with another lipophilic centrally acting β-blocker, seems to work quite well (18).

Akinesia is one of the more subtle forms of toxicity that antipsychotics can induce. It is characterized by diminished spontaneity with decreased speech, few gestures, apathy, and indifference. There is often a difficult three-way differential among drug-induced akinesia, postpsychotic depression, and undertreated schizophrenia with negative symptoms predominating. Here a

TABLE 2–5. **Agents for the treatment of extrapyramidal syndromes**

Generic name (by class)	Trade name	Usual dose	Comments
Anticholinergics			
Benztropine[a]	Cogentin	0.5–2 mg tid	1–2 mg iv for acute dystonia
Biperiden	Akineton	2 mg once a day to tid	
Procyclidine	Kemadrin	2.5–7.5 mg tid	
Trihexyphenidyl[a]	Artane	1–5 mg tid	2 mg iv for acute dystonia
Antihistamines			
Diphenhydramine[a]	Benadryl	12.5–50 mg tid or qid	25–50 mg iv for acute dystonia
β-Blockers			
Propranolol[a]	Inderal and others	10–20 mg tid or qid	The treatment of choice for akathisia; not indicated for other EPS

[a]Available generically.

careful history should help. If signs and symptoms are caused by undertreatment, then the symptoms should have been present all along. If they are present secondary to postpsychotic depression, then depressive cognition should be present. If the cause is the drug, then the symptoms should be dose dependent. In this case, they should be treated like any other EPS. Some clinicians argue that this is so ubiquitous and so difficult to diagnose that routine prophylactic antiparkinsonian treatment is required. Antiparkinsonian agents should not be reflexively used, but one should maintain a high index of suspicion and a low threshold for antiparkinsonian use.

Sedation is common with low-potency agents. At times sedation may be desired; at other times it is not. The patient frequently accommodates to sedation over time. This symptom correlates with antihistaminic effects.

Orthostatic hypotension correlates with a drug's blockade of the α-adrenergic receptor. Low-potency drugs are more likely to do this. This may be a dose-limiting factor, particularly with elderly patients. In measuring orthostasis it is best to measure blood pressure and pulse while the patient is sitting or lying, after standing, and again while still standing 5 minutes later. This should be correlated with a patient's complaints of lightheadedness or dizziness. Patients should be warned of this possibility and encouraged to get up slowly from squatting or from prolonged lying or sitting.

Anticholinergic side effects can be problematic for those drugs with high muscarinic affinity. These may include urinary retention, especially in patients with enlarged prostates; erectile and ejaculatory disturbances; visual blurring; and dry mouth. Dry mouth and blurred vision frequently improve with time.

Tardive Dyskinesia

Tardive dyskinesia remains a major source of concern. It is defined as abnormal, stereotypic, involuntary movements caused by exposure to prolonged dopamine blockade, as seen with antipsychotics.

It is thought that the receptor compensates by upregulating or increasing the number of dopamine receptors and also increasing the avidity with which the receptor seeks the transmitter.

Although buccolingual movements are the most common presentation, any muscle, including even the diaphragm, can be involved. Movements are classically choreoathetotic, but may involve tremor or more static posturing even to the point of dystonia. The movements disappear during sleep. Patients may be able to suppress them briefly. They will increase with stress. Movement elsewhere in the body, as with distracting maneuvers such as finger tapping, will increase the dyskinesia. The movements will initially get worse as the antipsychotic is withdrawn, but this is clearly the appropriate long-range strategy. Although increasing the dose will lead to short-term improvement as the upregulated receptors are blocked, the gain will be temporary because new receptors will begin to sprout. Thus the temporary solution afforded by increasing the dose of the antipsychotic will ultimately only escalate the problem.

Differential Diagnosis

The differential diagnosis is long and complicated. EPS can, at times, be difficult to distinguish from tardive dyskinesia. Decreasing the dose of the antipsychotic can help because EPS should improve and tardive dyskinesia should initially worsen. Schizophrenic patients postured and had involuntary movements long before antipsychotics were introduced. Finding unmedicated schizophrenic patients is difficult, but spontaneous dyskinesias are reported frequently among this population. The prevalence of both tardive and spontaneous dyskinesias will increase with age. Patients on neuroleptics may show involuntary movements when their drugs are abruptly withdrawn. This is termed *withdrawal dyskinesia* and may represent one of the earliest manifestations of the disorder. There are conflicting data about whether periodic withdrawal is helpful or harmful. Animal models suggest that periodic discontinuation may create more problems, but drug holidays clearly have diagnostic value because withdrawal dyskinesia should alert the physician to make every attempt possible to stop the medication.

All patients should be routinely monitored with a reliable rating instrument. The Abnormal Involuntary Movement Scale (AIMS) is the most widely used and is as good as any (Table 2–6). It can be filled out as the clinician interviews the patient. With practice it can be completed in several minutes.

Disagreement about diagnostic criteria accounts for some of the wide variability in the estimates of tardive dyskinesia incidence and prevalence, but the incidence is probably about 15% of patients with chronic neuroleptic exposure (19). It is similarly problematic to define the percentage of patients whose dyskinesias will clear with discontinuation of the drug. Probably between one-third and one-half of dyskinetic patients will not reverse even if made drug free. This is a frightening statistic that should make us reserve antipsychotics for patients who truly need them.

Tardive dystonia is in many respects like tardive dyskinesia, differing primarily in that it often involves younger patients and that it appears to be more common in men (20). Involuntary blepharospasm may be an early warning. This has been successfully treated with botulinum toxin (21).

Risk Factors

Certain risk factors should make the clinician particularly circumspect. Elderly patients are less likely to have a reversal of dyskinetic movements on discontinuation. Patients with affective disorders get far worse tardive dyskinesia and at an earlier age than do their congeners with schizophrenia (22). The clinician should not lose track of the tremendous good that neuroleptics can do, but they should be reserved for those patients who really need them. Intuitively it makes sense to prescribe antipsychotics at the lowest possible dose, but neither length of exposure, total exposure, use of anticholinergics, nor maximum dose have been clearly documented as risk factors.

TABLE 2–6. Abnormal Involuntary Movement Scale

1. Observe gait on the way into the room.
2. Have patient remove gum or dentures if ill fitting.
3. See if the patient is aware of any movements.
4. Have the patient sit on a firm chair without arms with his or her hands on his or her knees, legs slightly apart, and feet flat on the floor. Now and throughout the exam, look at the entire body for movements.
5. Have the patient sit with hands unsupported, dangling over the knees.
6. Ask patient to open his or her mouth twice. Look for tongue movements.
7. Ask patient to protrude his or her tongue twice.
8. Ask patient to tap thumb against each finger for 15 seconds with each hand. Observe face and legs.
9. Have patient stand with arms extended forward.

Rate each item on a 0–4 scale for the highest severity observed. Movements that occur only on activation merit 1 point less than those that occur spontaneously.

0 = none; 1 = minimal, may be extreme normal; 2 = mild;
3 = moderate; 4 = severe

Facial and oral movements

1. Muscles of facial expression	0	1	2	3	4
2. Lips and perioral area	0	1	2	3	4
3. Jaw	0	1	2	3	4
4. Tongue	0	1	2	3	4

Extremity movements

5. Upper	0	1	2	3	4
6. Lower	0	1	2	3	4

Trunk movements

7. Neck, shoulders, hips	0	1	2	3	4

Global judgments

8. Severity of abnormal movements	0	1	2	3	3
9. Incapacitation because of abnormal movements	0	1	2	3	4
10. Patient's awareness of abnormal movements	0	1	2	3	4

0 = Unaware   4 = Severe distress

Source. Modified from Guy W: *ECDEU Assessment Manual for Psychopharmacology.* Rockville, MD, US Department of Health, Education and Welfare, 1976.

Treatment

There is no proven treatment for tardive dyskinesia. Any therapy must therefore be regarded as experimental. The cornerstone should be discontinuation of the antipsychotic, but this should not be done reflexively. The decision whether or not to stop the drug presents a profound ethical dilemma. A judgment has to be made about whether the risk of worsening tardive dyskinesia is graver than the risk of worsening psychosis. This is a difficult dilemma and a choice that most therapists prefer not to make alone. Many patients have a kind of agnosia about the movements. They know that they are there because others have commented on them, but they themselves are not terribly concerned. The decision should be made by the patient if competent, and by the family if the patient is not, after receiving input from the physician.

If drug withdrawal is helpful, the results are usually apparent within the first 3–6 months. If the movements continue and if they are severe enough to require treatment, several alternatives can be investigated. Dopamine depleters have the advantage of having some antipsychotic efficacy. Dopamine depletion has not been associated with the onset of tardive dyskinesia, although depression and hypotension have been associated with the use of reserpine. Treatment is initiated with 0.25 mg/day, with similar daily increments, ultimately dividing the dose to four times per day. The maximal dose is about 6 mg/day. Orthostatic blood pressure should be monitored throughout the trial.

There is a reciprocal antagonism between striatal acetylcholine and dopamine. Increasing acetylcholine should therefore ameliorate tardive dyskinesia. Physostigmine, an inhibitor of cholinesterase that degrades acetylcholine, has proved helpful, but it is short acting and has to be given intravenously. Other cholinergic agonists are either toxic or ineffective. Although there are no data to indicate that anticholinergics cause tardive dyskinesia, they may worsen it, so they should be withdrawn if possible. γ-Aminobutyric acid (GABA) inhibits nigrostriatal dopamine activity. Benzodiazepines therefore have theoretical appeal, but they have to be used at such high doses as to be of no clinical utility. There is also preliminary support for α-tocopherol or vitamin E based on the theory that tardive dyskinesia might result from free-radical activity. Occasional patients respond to noradrenergic antagonists such as propranolol or clonidine (23).

In summary, tardive dyskinesia represents a condition that may or may not be reversible and for which there is no effective treatment. It is desirable to discontinue the antipsychotic if possible, but this decision should be reached by the patient and his or her family with input from the physician. The primary intervention should be preventive. Antipsychotics should be reserved for patients who truly need them. An explanation of the possibility of tardive dyskinesia should be made as soon as the patient's mental status has cleared sufficiently to offer true informed consent. Patients should be regularly assessed with the AIMS or a similar instrument, and periodic drug holidays should be attempted so as to provoke withdrawal dyskinesia.

Rarer Toxicities

Low-potency agents, such as chlorpromazine or thioridazine in particular, are thought to lower the seizure threshold. Molindone may pose somewhat less liability than other antipsychotics for seizure induction (24). When combining antipsychotics and anticonvulsants, clinicians should exercise caution because there is considerable potential for enzyme induction and consequent alteration of previously stable levels.

High doses of antipsychotics, particularly in young males, have been associated with *drug-induced catatonia*. If this is the case, the patient should improve if the drug is withdrawn or if an anticholinergic is added.

Antipsychotics *prolong ventricular repolarization*. Thioridazine is the most offensive, but this is generally a more theoretical than real problem. They also may be associated with an increased Q-R interval and T wave flattening.

Retrograde ejaculation can occur with thioridazine. *Increased appetite* and *weight gain* are not unusual. Molindone, for some reason, seems immune from this effect (25). *Galactorrhea* and *gynecomastia* can occur. They are associated with an increase in the prolactin level. Dopamine is thought to be prolactin-releasing inhibitory factor, so it is not surprising that prolactin levels increase and these effects eventuate. *Menstrual irregularities* are not infrequent. Patients should be warned that these medicines are not a reliable form of birth control.

Phenothiazines in particular have been associated with *hepatitis*. Liver biopsies show a cholestatic picture. This typically occurs early in the course of treatment. There is little evidence of cross-sensitivity with nonphenothiazine neuroleptics. *Agranulocytosis* has been very rare and typically occurs with low-potency drugs, but patients should have complete blood counts drawn at signs of infection. *Photosensitivity* is common with low-potency agents. Patients should be given sunscreens routinely. *Lenticular* and *corneal deposits* have been reported with phenothiazines. Thioridazine has led to pigmentary retinopathy at doses of 1 g/day. The Food and Drug Administration has, as a result, imposed a ceiling of 800 mg/day. Hypothalamic dysfunction may be associated with *poikilothermia*, or a loss of temperature regulation that causes a tendency toward hyperthermia in the summer and hypothermia in the winter. This is particularly likely in elderly patients. The *syndrome of inappropriate antidiuretic hormone* has been reported.

Neuroleptic-induced *supersensitivity psychosis* has been reported by Chouinard and Jones (26). They described patients who also had tardive dyskinesia and appeared to require escalating doses of neuroleptics to maintain the same effect. Missing a single dose or getting to the end of a depot cycle was associated with positive symptoms. This is thought to represent extension of dopaminergic hypersensitivity to the mesolimbic system, in addition to the neostriatal involvement associated with tardive dyskinesia.

Neuroleptic malignant syndrome (NMS) is a potentially lethal reaction to antipsychotics characterized by muscular rigidity, decreased level of consciousness, and autonomic dysfunction including hyperthermia, labile blood pressure, tachycardia, and diaphoresis (27). Laboratory findings include elevated creatinine phosphokinase and leukocytosis. It can occur either early or late in the course of neuroleptic treatment and is far more common with high-potency drugs. Fortunately, it is rare (28). Coprescription of lithium appears to be a risk factor. It has also been seen after the withdrawal of dopamine agonists. The differential is quite complicated. A clinically indistinguishable syndrome (Bell's mania) was described more than a hundred years before the first antipsychotic was developed (29). Patients need to have a full workup as for any fever of unknown origin. The fatality rate is approximately 15%. Various treatments have been suggested, including bromocriptine, carbidopa/levodopa, amantadine, and dantrolene.

Although it is not definite that aggressive treatment is helpful, it is certain that antipsychotics need to be discontinued and that supportive treatment with antipyretics, antihypertensives, antiarrythmics, and whatever other agents are necessary needs to be instituted (30). If rhabdomyolysis leads to renal failure, then dialysis may be necessary. Low-dose heparin may prevent pulmonary emboli in the NMS patient who may be immobilized. Dantrolene inhibits the release of intracellular calcium, thereby preventing heat generated by tonic muscular contraction. This has led to its use in malignant hyperthermia. It is used in doses of 0.8–2.5 mg/kg body weight every 6 hours in patients with NMS. Alternatively, dopamine agonists (amantadine 100 mg bid or bromocriptine 2.5–20 mg tid) are used on the basis of the theory that reduced dopaminergic function is the cause of NMS. Many patients who have had such treatments have improved, but some have died, and it is not clear that specific medical treatment alters the natural course of the disorder. Because controlled trials are virtually impossible with these patients, treatment needs to continue to be empirical.

Long-term management of the patient who has recovered from NMS poses major difficulties (31). If possible, conventional antipsychotics should be avoided because NMS can redevelop with subsequent dopamine blockade. If conventional antipsychotics must be reinstituted, it is wise to wait as long as possible after the acute episode. It is important that the patient be well hydrated. Low-potency antipsychotics should be used preferentially and at as low a dose as is possible. If a low-potency agent caused the NMS, one of a different class should be chosen. Coprescription of lithium should be avoided. Clozapine should be considered. Although NMS has been reported with clozapine use, it is unusual and it is not clear that clozapine alone can induce the syndrome.

■ INTERACTIONS

Drug-drug interactions with neuroleptics are largely predictable from each drug's receptor effects. Those compounds high on the spectrum of muscarinic affinity should not be combined with other anticholinergic agents. Drugs that are potent α-blockers should be monitored closely if combined with agents that promote orthostasis. Drugs that have significant standardized H_1 affinity pose a risk of excessive sedation if combined with other central nervous system depressants. A list of some of the more commonly encountered interactions is presented in Table 2–7.

■ DEPOT ANTIPSYCHOTICS

Most neuroleptics have half-lives of 24 hours or more. Thus they can ordinarily be prescribed each day at bedtime. Sedation is less of a problem, and compliance is enhanced by once-daily dosing. Longer-acting, or depot, antipsychotics have been developed in an attempt to further ensure adherence to a prescribed regimen.

Currently, three depot agents are available in the United States (Table 2–8). All are given parenterally and have the advantage of only needing to be given every 1–4 weeks. Compliance is ensured, and there is no worry about absorption. On the other hand, problems may take a long time to correct themselves. The drug half-lives are so long that it will take a considerable period to reach steady state and a similarly long time to wash out should there be difficulties.

These medications are appropriately reserved for patients with malabsorption of oral medication, demonstrated histories of noncompliance, marked ambivalence about medication, or prominent risk factors for drug defaulting, such as ego-syntonic delusional systems. With these patients, long-acting medications can make a dramatic difference. Depot agents are most typically used for the maintenance phase of treatment, but they can be used during

TABLE 2–7. **Antipsychotic interactions**

Interacting agent	Effect	Comments
Alcohol	Additive effect	Patients should be told that one drink may seem like several.
Barbiturates	Increase neuroleptic metabolism	
β-Blockers	Risk of orthostasis	
Bethanidine, guanadrel, guanethedine	Decreased antihypertensive effect	Uptake is blocked.
Carbamazepine	Decreases antipsychotic level	Clearest for haloperidol.
Levodopa	Decreased levodopa effect	Inhibits dopamine uptake.
Lithium	Increased incidence of NMS epidemiologically	Can be coprescribed but monitor for NMS.
NSAIDs	Extreme drowsiness	Reported with haloperidol and indomethacin.

Note. NMS = neuroleptic malignant syndrome; NSAIDs = nonsteroidal anti-inflammatory drugs.

the initial, nonacute phase as well. Their toxicities are those that would be expected for any high-potency neuroleptic.

Normative doses are 12.5–50 mg of fluphenazine decanoate every 1–3 weeks, or 25–150 mg of haloperidol decanoate every 3–5 weeks. Steady state will not be reached until approximately four times the half-life. Until that time, patients previously maintained on oral regimens should continue their oral agent with a gradual tapering while the depot level is climbing. The initial dose of the depot agent is difficult to estimate, but the usual factors, including size, age, and degree of psychosis and agitation, should be taken into account. Once an initial, preferably low-dose regimen has been achieved, both dose and duration will have to be adjusted. The two key questions are whether the peak dose is sufficient to offer antipsychotic effect and whether it is lasting long enough.

■ CLOZAPINE

Clozapine was patented 30 years ago and was extensively used in Europe until a sudden outbreak of agranulocytosis associated with its use was noted in 1975. This led to its withdrawal from the

TABLE 2–8. **Depot antipsychotic agents**

Compound	Dosage and interval	Approximate single-dose plasma half-life (days)	Approximate single-dose peak level obtained (days)
Fluphenazine decanoate[a]	12.5–50 mg every 1–3 weeks	7	1
Fluphenazine enanthate[a]	12.5–50 mg every 1–2 weeks	4	2
Haloperidol decanoate	25–150 mg every 3–5 weeks	21	7

[a]Available generically.

market and cessation of attempts to make it available in the United States. By this time it was clear that there was something quite unique about the medication and a suggestion that patients with schizophrenia who had failed to respond to conventional agents might improve with clozapine. Organizations such as the National Alliance for the Mentally Ill exerted continuous pressure to see that the drug was not abandoned. A large and well-developed protocol made it clear that there was something unique about clozapine and that careful monitoring could prevent enduring hematologic toxicity (32). Use of clozapine requires weekly monitoring of complete blood counts *for as long as the drug is prescribed.* The original plan demanded that all hematologic monitoring be done through a centralized laboratory. This was ultimately changed because it made this already costly medication prohibitively expensive. Financing remains a major issue because the cost of the medication approaches $5,000 annually and state Medicaid agencies are grappling with whether this treatment should be supported. From a purely monetary point of view, there is considerable rationale for doing so once the cost of inpatient hospitalization for treatment-refractory patients is factored in.

Clozapine differs from conventional antipsychotics because it only weakly blocks the D_2 receptor. It has almost equal affinity for the D_1 receptor. It has potent anticholinergic, antihistaminic, and α-blocking effects (33). Side effects are in many ways similar to those seen with classical low-potency antipsychotics. Sedation and fatigue are common, especially in the early stages of treatment. Weight gain can be severe and often plateaus at around 6 months of treatment. Surprisingly, given that it is a potent anticholinergic, there is a great deal of drooling, typically worst at night. Fever may be seen during the first few weeks of treatment. Because of the risk of agranulocytosis, there should be an immediate complete blood count; if this is within normal limits, the fever will typically reverse. Seizures may occur in a dose-related fashion: the incidence is 4.4% for doses of 600–900 mg/day, 2.7% for doses of 300–600 mg/day, and 1% for doses below 300 mg/day. Overly rapid escalation of dose may be a risk factor, as is history of head trauma or seizure disorder (34). If an anticonvulsant is to be coprescribed, it should not be carbamazepine because of worry about hematologically additive effects. Respiratory depression and even arrest have been reported rarely. There is a suggestion that coprescription of a benzodiazepine may increase vulnerability for this side effect.

Because clozapine minimally blocks the D_2 receptor, we would expect that it would not lead to EPS or NMS. There have been scattered reports connecting NMS with clozapine, but several of the reports do not seem to meet diagnostic criteria. EPS and tardive dyskinesia do not seem to occur. There is debate in the literature about whether clozapine actually treats tardive dyskinesia or whether it merely allows discontinuation of the offending agent. This is not clear, but it does seem definite that it will not cause dyskinesia.

The major problem of toxicity is agranulocytosis. This is an immune-mediated phenomenon occurring in patients exposed to clozapine at the rate of approximately 1%–2% annually. *Patients who have had clozapine-mediated agranulocytosis should never be reexposed to the drug.* Although 75% of cases occur during the first 6 months of exposure, *agranulocytosis can occur at any time and monitoring should, therefore, continue indefinitely.* The current treatment guidelines call for weekly complete blood counts for the duration of treatment, with increased scrutiny for any white blood cell count less than 3,500 and discontinuation of treatment for any white blood cell count less than 2,000 or any absolute granulocyte count less than 1,000. Patients discontinued from clozapine because of agranulocytosis should be seen immediately by a hematologist. Fortunately, there is no evidence of cross-reactivity with other psychotropic agents. The special risks of clozapine demand that full informed consent be obtained and that clozapine only be given to patients who can comply with weekly blood testing.

Most of the clinical trials with clozapine were conducted with patients who failed to respond to multiple trials of conventional antipsychotics, which were then used as comparison agents. Thus the deck was stacked against the usual medications. What has emerged is very clear evidence that clozapine will help a substantial number of patients who do not respond to more usual compounds. There have been claims that this is a "superior antipsychotic." This is largely without substantiation, and it could be better phrased that it is a superior antipsychotic for those patients who do not respond to conventional D_2 antagonists.

There have been debates about whether clozapine preferentially attacks negative symptoms. This is not clear, but there is considerable evidence that it can affect both positive and negative symptoms in some patients.

Who then should receive clozapine? It should never be used as a first-line antipsychotic. It can, however, offer substantial benefit to patients who do not respond to conventional agents or who are intolerant of them. All of the controlled studies in the literature have been with patients with schizophrenia, but there are suggestions that it may have a role in patients with psychotic affective disorders who are intolerant of or unresponsive to conventional antipsychotics (35).

Typically clozapine is begun with 12.5 mg/day or bid and then increased, using tid dosing, by 25–50 mg/day for 2–3 days. The maximum allowable dose is 900 mg/day, although it is unusual to require more than 450 mg/day. Because the hematologic risk continues indefinitely, it is not wise to continue the medication for more than 3 months in the absence of signs of response.

■ REFERENCES

1. Dubin WR, Weiss KJ, Dorn JM: Pharmacotherapy of psychiatric emergencies. J Clin Psychopharmacol 6:210–222, 1986
2. Salzman C, Solomon D, Miyawa K, et al: Parenteral lorazepam versus parenteral haloperidol for the control of psychotic disruptive behavior. J Clin Psychiatry 52:177–180, 1991
3. Altamura AC, Mauri MC, Mantero M, et al: Clonazepam/

haloperidol combination therapy in schizophrenics—double blind study. Acta Psychiatr Scand 76:702–706, 1987

4. Overall JE, Gorham DR: The Brief Psychiatric Rating Scale. Psychol Rep 10:799–812, 1962

5. Rifkin A, Doddi S, Karajgi B, et al: Dosage of haloperidol for schizophrenia. Arch Gen Psychiatry 48:166–179, 1991

6. Van Putten T, Marder SR, Mintz J: A controlled dose comparison of haloperidol in newly admitted schizophrenic patients. Arch Gen Psychiatry 47:754–758, 1990

7. Baldessarini RJ, Cohen BM, Teicher MH: Significance of neuroleptic dose and plasma level in the pharmacological treatment of psychoses. Arch Gen Psychiatry 45:79–91, 1988

8. Goff DC, Henderson DC, Amico E: Cigarette smoking in schizophrenia: relationship to psychopathology and medication side effects. Am J Psychiatry 149:1189–1194, 1992

9. Van Putten T, Marder S, Wirshing WC, et al: Neuroleptic plasma levels. Schizophr Bull 17:197–216, 1991

10. Christison GW, Kirch DG, Wyatt RJ: When symptoms persist: choosing among alternative somatic treatments for schizophrenia. Schizophr Bull 17:217–245, 1991

11. Linden R, Davis JM, Rubinstern J: High vs. low dose treatment with antipsychotic agents. Psychiatric Annals 12:769–781, 1982

12. Bellack AS, Mueser KT: Psychosocial treatment for schizophrenia. Schizophr Bull 19:317–361, 1993

13. Jeste DV, Caligiuri MD: Tardive dyskinesia. Schizophr Bull 19:303–315, 1993

14. Schooler NR: Maintenance medicine for schizophrenia. Schizophr Bull 17:311–324, 1991

15. Kroessler D: Relative efficacy rates for therapies of delusional depression. Convulsive Therapy 1:173–182, 1985

16. Raskind MA, Risse SC, Lampe TH: Dementia and antipsychotic drugs. J Clin Psychiatry 48 (suppl 5):16–18, 1987

17. Opler LA, Feinberg SS: The role of pimozide in clinical psychiatry: a review. J Clin Psychiatry 52:221–233, 1991

18. DuPuis B, Catteau J, Dumon JP, et al: Comparison of propran-

olol, sotalol, and betaxolol in the treatment of neuroleptic-induced akathisia. Am J Psychiatry 144:802–805, 1987

19. Kane JM, Smith JM: Tardive dyskinesia: prevalence and risk factors. Arch Gen Psychiatry 39:473–481, 1982

20. Wojci JD, Falk WE, Fink JS, et al: A review of 32 cases of tardive dystonia. Am J Psychiatry 148:1055–1059, 1991

21. Truong DD, Hermanowicz N, Rontal M: Botulinum toxin in treatment of tardive dyskinetic syndrome. J Clin Psychopharmacol 10:438–439, 1990

22. Yassa R, Nastase C, Dupont D, et al: Tardive dyskinesia in elderly psychiatric patients: a 5-year study. Am J Psychiatry 149:1206–1211, 1992

23. American Psychiatric Association: Tardive Dyskinesia: A Task Force Report of the American Psychiatric Association. Washington, DC, American Psychiatric Association, 1992

24. Oliver AP, Luchins DJ, Wyatt RJ: Neuroleptic-induced seizures: an in vitro technique for assessing relative risk. Arch Gen Psychiatry 39:206–209, 1982

25. Doss FW: The effect of antipsychotic drugs on body weight. J Clin Psychiatry 40:528–530, 1979

26. Chouinard G, Jones BD: Neuroleptic-induced supersensitivity psychosis: clinical and pharmacological characteristics. Am J Psychiatry 137:16–21, 1980

27. Lazarus A, Mann SC, Caroff SN: The Neuroleptic Malignant Syndrome and Related Conditions. Washington, DC, American Psychiatric Press, 1989

28. Gelenberg AJ, Bellinghausen B, Wojcik JD, et al: A prospective study of neuroleptic malignant syndrome in a short-term psychiatric hospital. Am J Psychiatry 145:517–518, 1988

29. Bell LV: On a form of disease resembling some advanced stages of mania and fever. Am J Insanity, October 1849, pp 97–127

30. Levenson JL: Neuroleptic malignant syndrome. Am J Psychiatry 142:1137–1145, 1985

31. Lazarus A, Caroff SN, Mann SC: Beyond NMS: management after the acute episode. Psychiatric Annals 21:165–174, 1991

32. Kane J, Honigfeld G, Singer J, et al: Clozapine for the treatment resistant schizophrenic: a double blind comparison with chlorpromazine. Arch Gen Psychiatry 45:789–796, 1988

33. Baldessarini RJ, Frankenberg FR: Clozapine: a novel antipsychotic agent. N Engl J Med 324:746–754, 1991

34. Devinsky O, Honigfeld G, Patin J: Clozapine-related seizures. Neurology 41:369–371, 1991

35. McElroy SL, Dessain EC, Pope HG, et al: Clozapine in the treatment of psychotic mood disorders, schizoaffective disorder, and schizophrenia. J Clin Psychiatry 52:411–414, 1991

ANTIDEPRESSANTS

■ HISTORY

By 1953 there were suggestions that iproniazid, a monoamine oxidase inhibitor (MAOI) used for the treatment of tuberculosis, had antidepressant properties. Until then stimulants and electroconvulsive therapy (ECT) were the only biological treatments for depression. Further progress was made with the discovery of imipramine in 1957; the effects were so clear that Roland Kuhn knew he had an important new agent by the time the third patient had taken the drug. Because chlorpromazine was discovered at approximately the same time, there was great hope for a pharmacological cure of mental illness. We remain considerably short of that goal, but there is little question that antidepressants are a very significant addition.

The recently arrived serotonin-specific reuptake inhibitors (SSRIs), including fluoxetine, sertraline, and paroxetine, offer no improvement in terms of efficacy or rapidity of onset, but they do have different side-effect profiles. For the purposes of our discussion, we will include SSRIs and atypical agents such as bupropion and trazodone with the second-generation antidepressants.

■ TARGET SYMPTOMS

In Chapter 1 it was emphasized that antidepressants do not treat depression, but rather the vegetative signs associated with the syndrome. Table 3–1 highlights the distinction between the targets for psychotherapy and for the biological therapy of depression. The important point is that the two treatments are additive (1). Medication will help with the hopelessness and the anergia that make psychological interventions virtually impossible with a deeply depressed patient. A solid relationship with a patient will, in turn, reinforce medication compliance and increase the likelihood of having sufficient information to make rational pharmacological choices.

The vegetative signs include sleep interruption, particularly early morning awakening; anorexia with weight loss; constipation; psychomotor changes; diurnal variation (with mood worse in the morning); and diminished libido. It should be noted that this description reasonably approximates the DSM-IV definition of melancholia (2). Symptoms such as guilt, anhedonia (absence of pleasure), anergia (diminished energy), hopelessness, and helplessness may also respond to antidepressants but are not as robust predictors of good response to medication.

The typical, but not invariable, pattern of improvement is for signs to respond before symptoms. Patients should be forewarned about this possibility because this information may encourage them to remain in treatment. Others will notice a change before the patient is aware of it; humor may return before mood, sleep may normalize several days before guilt feelings diminish. Many toxicities are immediate, whereas the antidepressant effect often takes several weeks. Seriously depressed patients are also often imbued with a profound sense of hopelessness that leaves them certain that nothing can help. Unless directly addressed, these issues often result in drug default.

TABLE 3–1. **Effects of psychotherapy and somatic therapy in depression**

Therapy	Signs and symptoms relieved	Time course
Psychotherapy	Mood, suicidal ideation, work, interests, guilt, social adjustment	4–8 weeks
Somatic therapy	Vegetative symptoms, especially sleep and appetite disturbance	1–3 weeks

Source. From DiMascio A, Weissman MM, Prosoff BA, et al: "Differential Symptom Reduction by Drugs and Psychotherapy in Acute Depression." *Archives of General Psychiatry* 36:1450–1456, 1979.

■ CONTRAINDICATIONS

One must always rule out the "organic" causes of depression; that is, depression secondary to other disease processes. Any good basic psychiatry text will furnish you with a long list of illnesses and toxicities to be considered. A less than exhaustive discussion of some of the more common etiologies follows.

Always consider the possibility of a toxic reaction to medication or other exogenous substance. The key step is to review medication and drug intake in an attempt to correlate them with the onset of the depression. Reserpine, clonidine, and methyldopa are often associated with depression; lipophilic β-blockers may be as well. Central nervous system depressants, notably barbiturates and benzodiazepines, are potential offenders as well. Withdrawal from stimulants can be problematic.

Carcinoma of any type, but especially of the pancreas, can present with depression. Dementia, irrespective of etiology, can manifest depression before overt cognitive impairment. Almost any systemic infection can do this as well.

A wide variety of metabolic and endocrine disorders can result in the syndrome. Thyroid abnormality, especially hypothyroidism, is frequently associated with depression. The same can be said for adrenal dysfunction, hyperparathyroidism, diabetes, and vitamin B_{12} and folate deficiencies. These illnesses serve to underscore the importance of a good review of systems.

It should be remembered that sadness is not the same as depression. It is, instead, one feature of a syndrome; some patients may lack depressed mood and instead present with irritability. By the same token, the presence of a significant stressor should not necessarily dissuade you from using an antidepressant (see the discussion of adjustment disorder with depressed mood).

Caution should be exercised in patients with histories of mania either in themselves or in family members. Any antidepressant treatment has the potential of cycling a depressed patient into mania. Patients with significant risk factors should probably have lithium prophylaxis along with the antidepressant.

Medical contraindications are primarily cardiac and are discussed in the section on toxicity.

■ INDICATIONS

Depression

Major Depression, Recurrent or Single Episode

The vegetative signs previously discussed remain the most important predictors of response. The efficacy of antidepressants in this disorder is clear. The usual figures quoted are that depression will resolve in 50% of patients within 6 weeks with no treatment, 55% with placebo, 65% with an MAOI, 70% with a heterocyclic antidepressant (HCA), and 85%–90% with ECT. Many believe that these response percentages for active treatment are low and are higher if thorough and aggressive therapy is provided. The figures would also improve if the studies were limited to patients with melancholia. Other positive predictors are intuitively obvious: personal or even family history of response to medication, and good premorbid or intermorbid functioning. The impressive response to no treatment or placebo serves to remind us that acute depression is often a self-limiting illness and that medications will, at times, do no more than accelerate the resolution of the process.

Some common errors to avoid:

1. *Thinking that a little bit of depression merits a little bit of drug.* If you are going to treat, then nothing less than a full therapeutic dose should be used. To do otherwise merely exposes the patient to toxicity without the opportunity for benefit.
2. *Not treating for a long-enough period.* All antidepressant treatments take 2–3 weeks to work. Unfortunately, this process cannot be accelerated. Do not give up on an agent unless it has had at least 3 weeks at the appropriate dose without indication

of response. By the same token, once effective, antidepressants should not be discontinued prematurely. A National Institute of Mental Health collaborative study indicates that they should be continued for 16–20 weeks after a patient is completely free of symptoms (3). These suggestions still make sense for a patient recovering from a first episode, but recent data indicate that patients maintained on antidepressants for 3 years after the index episode are still at significantly greater risk for relapse if they are placed on placebo than if they continue with medication (4). Then patients with recurrent depressions should have their medication continued for long periods, perhaps even chronically.

3. *Missing the presence of psychotic features.* The rate of response for depression with psychotic features is greatest for ECT, followed by antidepressants combined with antipsychotics, followed by antipsychotics alone, and then antidepressants alone (5). These patients should be treated with a combination of an antipsychotic and an antidepressant or with ECT in the acute phase. Because there is evidence that patients with affective disorders are peculiarly vulnerable to tardive dyskinesia, every effort should be made to get them off the antipsychotic as quickly as can be done safely.

The decision about continuation of treatment depends on the following:

1. How predictable are the episodes?
2. Will the patient be able to seek treatment rapidly if symptoms recur?
3. How much warning does the patient have before getting into serious difficulty?

Patients who become suicidal early in the course of an episode should be treated more aggressively than patients who have several weeks of early morning awakening as a prodrome. Patients who become overwhelmed with hopelessness and are therefore less likely to engage in treatment should also have more extended prophylaxis. It is important that every effort be made to prevent relapse because repeat episodes are associated with a significant chance of developing into chronicity (6).

Bipolar Disorder, Depressed Phase

Treatment of the depressed phase of bipolar disorder illustrates the need to distinguish between treatment of an acute episode and prophylaxis. Lithium and carbamazepine are very effective agents for preventing the return of either depression or mania, but both are relatively ineffective in the treatment of a depressive episode. Patients with bipolar disorder in the depressed phase should be treated as unipolar depressed patients, differing only in that antidepressants or ECT pose the risk of inducing a manic episode. Depressed patients who have manic episodes induced by biological treatment are said to have type II bipolar disorder. Patients with personal or family history of mania are especially vulnerable. Patients with previous history of antidepressant-induced mania should have lithium or carbamazepine coadministered with the antidepressant. Other patients at risk warrant at least a watchful eye for the development of mania.

Dysthymia

There is surprisingly little literature about pharmacological approaches to dysthymia. What there is suggests that the response is significantly less robust than that seen with major depression, but that there is sufficient likelihood to warrant attempts at treatment. There is some suggestion that MAOIs might have a greater likelihood of benefit (7).

Adjustment Disorder With Depressed Mood

Formerly a distinction was made between "reactive" and "endogenous" depression. This terminology, fortunately, is entering into disuse. The key concept is that the predictors described earlier hold true whether the depression is secondary to a major loss or occurs without clear precipitating events. Many individuals recently widowed will have diminished appetite and libido, insomnia, and depressed mood. Acutely, this is a perfectly appropriate part of the grieving process, and these patients should obviously not be medicated. There can come a point, however, when the grieving process has gone on too long and no resolution appears to be forthcoming. This is the time when antidepressants have a role—not to make the grief disappear, but to facilitate the necessary mourning that will allow the patient to resume his or her life. The art is in deciding when this point has been reached. There is no exact answer to this question.

Atypical Depression

MAOIs may be helpful for the same depressive indications as are HCAs. In addition, they have been advocated in a wide variety of "atypical" depressions. These various syndromes all seem to have significant anxiety as a common feature. Reversed biological signs also often are cited, as is "reactivity of mood," which is the retained ability to have one's mood respond to environmental change. Studies have evaluated four predictors of MAOI response and found that the presence of any of the following symptoms make the likelihood of response to an MAOI greater than that to a tricyclic antidepressant (8, 9): increased appetite or weight when depressed, oversleeping or more time in bed when depressed, rejection sensitivity throughout adulthood, and severe fatigue creating a sense of leaden paralysis or extreme heaviness in arms or legs when depressed.

Panic Disorder

The pharmacological treatment of panic disorder is discussed in Chapter 8. MAOIs, certain atypical benzodiazepines, and all HCAs that have been studied, with the exception of trazodone and bupropion, have proved effective in preventing panic attacks.

Obsessive-Compulsive Disorder

Clomipramine and fluoxetine are peculiarly effective with obsessive-compulsive patients. This is discussed in more detail in Chapter 8.

Chronic Pain Syndromes

Low doses of antidepressants can be used both as adjuncts to analgesics and for a more direct analgesic effect. This is discussed in Chapter 8.

Eating Disorders

Patients with bulimia, but not with restrictive anorexia, appear to respond to both HCA and MAOI antidepressants. This is discussed in more detail in Chapter 8.

Substance Abuse

Antidepressants can facilitate withdrawal from cocaine. Data are more conflicting in studies done with alcoholic patients. Both topics are covered in more detail in Chapter 8.

Seasonal Affective Disorder

Some patients develop a pattern of recurrent wintertime depressions. These often resemble atypical depressions with anergia, hypersomnolence, and hyperphagia as prominent features. This syndrome, known as seasonal affective disorder, has proved to be responsive to bright light phototherapy (10). Standard pharmacological approaches such as use of MAOIs or HCAs have not been investigated, but clinical experience suggests that they are reasonable alternatives to the lights for patients who do not respond or who are unwilling or unable to manage phototherapy protocols.

■ BASIC PHARMACOLOGY

Heterocyclics

The HCAs include tetra-, tri-, bi-, and unicyclic antidepressants, distinguished by the number of rings in their chemical structures.

There is as much as a 10-fold variation in steady-state plasma levels among individuals. This is primarily due to variation in hepatic microenzyme activity, which is largely determined genetically. The drugs are well absorbed after oral administration and are tightly bound to α_1-glycoproteins and albumin. Because only free, unbound drug permeates the blood-brain barrier and is therefore psychoactive, minor changes in these plasma proteins can have a major impact. The α_1-glycoproteins are said to be stress related, with an increase noted with physical illness or other stress. Although there are theoretical reasons to think that the amount of free, or active, drug would decline in the face of stress, there is no clinically meaningful documentation of such an effect.

Plasma tricyclic levels reflect the total amount of drug, bound and unbound, and therefore may not always predict clinical efficacy (Table 3–2). Patients with atypical binding may well be outliers who respond at "nontherapeutic" blood levels. Nonethe-

TABLE 3–2. **Tricyclic plasma levels**

Advantages	Disadvantages

1. There are good data correlating level and response for three drugs:
  a. Imipramine—total for imipramine plus desipramine > 225 ng/ml
  b. Desipramine > 125 ng/ml
  c. Nortriptyline 50–150 ng/ml
2. For unresponsive or unusually toxic patients, levels allow determination of appropriate dosing.
	1. There are conflicting data for all other heterocyclic antidepressants.
	2. These data are for populations only. Any given patient could be an outlier.
	3. It is a technically difficult assay. Know your lab.

less, blood plasma level measurements can be quite helpful in arriving at the appropriate doses for some of these drugs.

The technique for determining a plasma level is relatively simple. Blood should be obtained 12 hours after the last dose in order to reflect trough values. Levels should not be drawn on a patient who is doing well; if, for some reason, this was done, the clinician should be guided by the patient's course and not the numbers. If a patient fails to respond or manifests significant toxicity, plasma levels can be of great value.

For nortriptyline there is convincing evidence of a "therapeutic window." The dose-response curve is curvilinear, so having too high a level is just as likely to be associated with nonresponse as having too low a level. The remaining two drugs for which there are good data, imipramine and desipramine, have linear responses; a plasma level anywhere above the threshold will be associated with response, although overshooting by too wide a margin will increase the likelihood of toxicity. Most laboratories will quote "therapeutic" levels for a number of other HCAs, but considerable skepticism should be invoked because data on all other compounds are quite conflicting (11).

Second-Generation Antidepressants

Several SSRIs are now available in the United States. These medications act by preventing the reuptake of serotonin into the presynaptic neuron leading to more serotonin being available in the synaptic cleft. They differ from one another primarily in terms of half-life.

Bupropion is a unique antidepressant whose mechanism of action is largely unknown. It does not affect the usual amines, but does lead to some release of dopamine.

These atypical antidepressants pose no advantage in terms of efficacy or rapidity of onset. Their side-effect profile is different and typically more benign. They are significantly more expensive than older HCAs. Most of the published data have focused on outpatients, and there is less information on their use with significantly depressed inpatients. There are no good data correlating blood levels and response for any of these medications.

Mechanism of Action

Even if patients are given appropriate doses, there will still be a 2- to 3-week lag time before the antidepressant effect will be evident. The delay in response is, unfortunately, shared by all biological treatments for depression. This leads to speculation about the mechanism of action of antidepressant treatments.

The old biogenic amine theory held that depression reflected decreased levels of norepinephrine and serotonin (5-hydroxytryptamine, or 5-HT) and that mania reflected an increase in these two neurotransmitters. Antidepressants were seen as effective because they blocked reuptake of these transmitters, leading to increased amounts of both. This thesis suffers from two flaws: 1) certain atypical, but effective, antidepressants do not block reuptake of norepinephrine and 5-HT, and 2) it does not account for the latency of response. Moreover, although most antidepressants do increase norepinephrine and 5-HT, they do so acutely, well before any effect is clinically apparent, so some other explanation must be invoked.

No single theory satisfactorily explains all antidepressant therapies. It may, in fact, be that drug X operates differently from drug Y, but certain generalities probably hold true. The lag time between initial administration and response is consistent with the time required to alter receptor sensitivity. Chronic, but not acute, administration of any biological antidepressant therapy will be associated with decreased sensitivity (downregulation) of the β-adrenergic receptor. This would seem a sufficient explanation were it not for its lack of specificity: chlorpromazine and amphetamine have the same effect and are not terribly helpful in the treatment of depression. Long-term, but not acute, treatment seems to be associated with upregulation of the postsynaptic α_1-receptor and desensitization of the inhibitory, autoregulatory, presynaptic α_2-receptor. The net result is the release of more norepinephrine per impulse and increased impact at the effector receptor. There seems to be a parallel process at the 5-HT receptor as well (12). It well may be that different antidepressants operate by different mechanisms and that this accounts for some patients' response to one antidepressant but not to another.

At one point, the latter view was widely held and patients were routinely tried on a serotonergic drug or an adrenergic drug, then switched to the other class if the first failed. Various lists order drugs as to serotonergic and adrenergic activity, but reality is less pure. Amitriptyline is usually noted as primarily serotonergic, yet its metabolite, nortriptyline, is considerably more adrenergic and the ratio of the two compounds in vivo will vary considerably. There still may be some rationale for such a switch, but it usually makes more sense to try a more radically different approach, such as lithium augmentation, an atypical antidepressant, an MAOI, or ECT.

Monoamine Oxidase Inhibitors

The MAOIs act through inactivation of the outer mitochondrial enzyme monoamine oxidase. Although the plasma half-lives of MAOIs are measured in hours, their biological half-lives are for weeks. This reflects the fact that they will continue to exert an influence until the enzyme has had time to regenerate, which will typically take 2 weeks, although isolated case reports imply that the impact can be a month or more for some. This represents one of the great problems with MAOIs: when they are unsuccessful the clinician's hands are tied for a long time. Patients must be off the drug for at least 2 weeks before it is safe to try either ECT or a heterocyclic. Work is being conducted in an attempt to find a substance that will block the enzyme, yet reverse readily. There will be considerably greater flexibility and safety once such drugs are available.

There are two types of monoamine oxidase, *MAO-A* and *MAO-B*. Distinctions between the two are relative and not absolute. MAO-A deaminates serotonin, norepinephrine, and epinephrine. MAO-B acts on dopamine. Experimental agents, such as clorgyline, that primarily affect MAO-A are more effective antidepressants than those like pargyline, which preferentially inhibit MAO-B. The usual MAOIs used as antidepressants are nonselective and affect both subtypes. Both MAO-A and MAO-B cleave tyramine and tryptamine. Tyramine is a potent pressor that is normally inactivated by MAO in the gut. If the enzyme is blocked and tyramine is ingested, there is the risk of hypertensive crisis. It is for this reason that patients on these drugs must be on a tyramine-free diet (13).

At one time, there was considerable enthusiasm about platelet MAO activity, based on the theory that this was an easily accessible reflection of the enzyme's activity in the brain. There is some crude correlation with phenelzine's antidepressant activity increasing with 85% or more inhibition of platelet MAO activity. The limitations of this approach may reflect the fact that platelet MAO activity is MAO-B, whereas most of the antidepressant effect reflects inhibition of MAO-A.

One advantage of MAOIs is their relative selectivity. They are essentially devoid of effect on the muscarinic receptor and are therefore frequently used with patients who are sensitive to anticholinergic toxicities. The lack of cholinergic impact is also shared with trazodone, fluoxetine, paroxetine, sertraline, and bupropion, as is an absence of effect on cardiac conduction. They are also unlikely to induce arrhythmia. The usual dose-limiting factor is orthostasis, probably secondary to an effect on α-adrenergic receptors.

■ DOSE AND DURATION OF TREATMENT

The most common error is prescribing inadequate amounts of these drugs for an inadequate period. Subtherapeutic doses expose patients to potential toxicity without the opportunity for benefit;

treating for less than 3–4 weeks often leads to prematurely abandoning a potentially helpful agent.

For HCAs there is as much as a 10-fold difference in dose and plasma level among individual patients. Table 3–3 lists normative doses, but it must be realized that many patients fall outside of these ranges. It is for this reason that drugs that have good data correlating plasma level and response are to be preferred. Particular note also should be taken of the compounds with atypical doses: nortriptyline and protriptyline are more potent than most, amoxapine and trazodone less potent. The second-generation antidepressants must be considered separately. Normally, all HCAs can be given at bedtime. Trazodone may need to be split during the day because of its very short plasma half-life. Large doses at bedtime can occasionally be accompanied by nightmares; if this is the case, the dose should be split. Single nighttime doses can also be a problem for the patient who gets up suddenly during the night to go to the bathroom because orthostasis can pose a difficulty. All HCAs, with the exception of protriptyline (which should be given in the morning), are typically sedating. Prescription at night is an example of attempting to benefit from toxicity.

A patient should be started on an HCA gradually. If a full treatment dose is begun right away, both the α_2 and anticholinergic toxicities may be more than the patient can tolerate. It usually makes sense to start the patient with 50 mg of imipramine or equivalent and increase by a similar quantity every 3–4 days. The dose can then be held at 150 or 200 mg, depending on the patient's size and tolerance for another 1–2 weeks in order to monitor response.

A reasonable guideline for dosage of phenelzine is to aim for 1 mg/kg of body weight. The usual range is 45–90 mg/day. Tranylcypromine may be considered twice as potent. Both drugs, but particularly tranylcypromine, are usually mildly activating. For this reason they should be taken in the morning, typically in a split dose. The dose should be gradually increased in much the same fashion as HCAs.

TABLE 3–3. **Heterocyclic antidepressants**

Generic name (by class)	Brand name	Half-life (hours)	Usual dose (mg)	Therapeutic plasma level (ng/ml)	Comments
Tertiary tricyclics[a]					
Amitriptyline[a]	Elavil, Endep, others	15	150–300	Controversial	Very sedating and very anticholinergic.
Clomipramine	Anafranil	32	150–250	Unknown	Very anticholinergic compound that inhibits reuptake of serotonin. Strong support for its use in obsessive-compulsive disorder.
Doxepin[a]	Adapin, Sinequan	17	150–300	Controversial	Quite sedating.
Imipramine[a]	Tofranil, SK-Pramine, Janimine, others	22	150–300	Total imipramine plus desipramine >225	The original tricyclic.
Trimipramine[a]	Surmontil	9	150–300	Unknown	Very sedating but little anticholinergic effect.
Secondary tricyclics[a]					
Desipramine[a]	Norpramin	21	150–300	>125	First-pass metabolite of imipramine.
Nortriptyline[a]	Aventyl, Pamelor	27	75–150	50–150	First-pass metabolite of amitriptyline.
Protriptyline	Vivactil	78	10–40	Unknown	The most activating heterocyclic.

TABLE 3–3. **Heterocyclic antidepressants** *(continued)*

Generic name (by class)	Brand name	Half-life (hours)	Usual dose (mg)	Therapeutic plasma level (ng/ml)	Comments
Dibenzoxazepine[a] Amoxapine[a]	Asendin	30	100–400	Unknown	Blocks dopamine receptors and has risk of tardive dyskinesia, extrapyramidal symptoms, and galactorrhea.
Tetracyclic Maprotiline[a]	Ludiomil	47	150–300	Unknown	Increased incidence of seizures; 3% develop a skin rash.
Triazolopyridine[a] Trazodone[a]	Desyrel	5	100–600	Unknown	Sedating; does not extend conduction deficits; does increase ventricular ectopy and cause priapism; safe overdoses.

Serotonin-specific reuptake inhibitors					
Fluoxetine	Prozac	72	10–40	Unknown	Pure serotonergic drug; does not interact with alcohol; weight *loss* noted; little orthostasis; somewhat activating.
Sertraline	Zoloft	25	50–200	Unknown	Approved January 1992. Shares many properties with fluoxetine.
Paroxetine	Paxil	24	20–40	Unknown	Approved January 1993. It may cause less anxiety than fluoxetine.
Aminoketones Bupropion	Wellbutrin	10	300–450	Unknown	Contraindicated in patients with a history of seizure or eating disorder.

[a] Available generically.

The typical dose for fluoxetine with depressed patients is 20 mg/day. Many patients will do well with even less. There is a liquid preparation available; alternatively, patients can be instructed to shake the contents of the 20-mg capsule into fruit juice, shake, and drink the appropriate portion, refrigerating the remainder. Patients may, on occasion, require 40 mg/day, but it is unusual to need more than that for depression. Sertraline is new to the market. The one fixed-dose study, which was quite compromised by small numbers, suggests that 50 mg/day may suffice (14). The pricing is such that patients may be better off splitting a 100-mg tablet in half rather than taking a 50-mg tablet. Bupropion use is limited by a dose-related increase in seizure frequency. As a result, the maximum allowable dose is 450 mg/day with no more than 150 mg to be taken at one time. The usual strategy is to begin with 100 mg bid, to increase the dose after several days to 100 mg tid, and to wait several weeks to see if that dose is effective before increasing it further.

The very long half-life of fluoxetine can be a problem if it needs to be discontinued. Five weeks should elapse before an MAOI should be instituted and tricyclics should be prescribed only cautiously and at low doses because their plasma levels (especially desipramine) may be significantly elevated (15).

For both MAOIs and HCAs there must be a minimum of 3–4 weeks (and often trials as long as 8–10 weeks are warranted) at an adequate dose before they should be considered a failure. If after a 3- to 4-week period there are early signs of response, the drug should be continued because it often takes 6 weeks for the maximal response to be evident.

The risk of relapse is greatest in the first several months after discontinuation of antidepressants. Because of this it is probably prudent to continue antidepressant therapy for a patient recovering from a first episode of depression for 16–20 weeks after he or she is symptom free (3). For patients with bipolar disease, lithium has been shown to have superior prophylactic efficacy over HCAs. For patients with unipolar disease, the results are comparable. In the presence of a family history of bipolar disorder, lithium is preferred; absent such a history, the physician would be wise to opt for whichever agent would lead to enhanced compliance. Recurrent patients should have medication maintained for several times their average cycle length before it is withdrawn (16). Data indicating risk for relapse 5 years after a depressive episode suggest that patients with recurrent depression should consider very long-term maintenance (4). It was once thought that maintenance doses should be lower than doses used for acute treatment. Recent data indicate that patients maintained on full antidepressant doses have less chance of relapse (17).

■ SIDE EFFECTS

HCAs, atypical antidepressants, and MAOIs share certain toxicities, some peculiar to a given class and some limited to certain agents within each group. Most antidepressants share a relatively low therapeutic index. All of them can be used to commit *suicide*. Because patients with depression are at high risk, some physicians avoid prescription of the very agents that could be of help to them. Such a blanket prohibition is not warranted, but patients should be routinely asked about suicidal ideation. Except in unusual situations, prescriptions should not be written for more than a 1-week supply with patients who have any thoughts of suicide. Admittedly, patients can cache away several weeks' worth, but writing a limited supply prevents impulsive acting out and forces the physician to reevaluate the patient frequently. Particular caution should be exercised when patients are starting to emerge from an episode. This is when suicide potential often maximizes, probably reflecting the asynchrony of response to antidepressants; energy often responds before suicidal ideation, leaving patients able to act.

There is renewed debate about whether biological treatment of depression carries the risk of inducing *mania*. Clearly, some patients who are receiving antidepressant therapy cycle into manic episodes. What is less clear is whether this happens more often than would occur without any intervention. The data on this are conflicting, but some individuals do cycle as a result of treatment and should have lithium or carbamazepine prophylaxis. Patients are at particular risk by virtue of past history of mania, family history of mania, or previous episodes of drug-induced cycling.

Heterocyclic Antidepressant Side Effects

Understanding which receptors are affected will go a long way toward predicting toxicities associated with particular agents.

TABLE 3–4. **Antidepressants and receptors**

Generic name	Anticholinergic affinity	α_1 affinity	H_1 affinity
Amitriptyline	4	3	3
Amoxapine	1	2	1
Bupropion[a]	0	0	0
Clomipramine	2	—	0
Desipramine	1	1	0
Doxepin	2	3	4
Fluoxetine	0	1/0	0
Imipramine	2	1	1
Maprotiline	1	1	2
Nortriptyline	1	1	1
Paroxetine	0	0	0
Protriptyline	3	1	0
Sertraline	0	0	0
Trazodone	0	2	0
Trimipramine	2	3	4

Note. 0 = no effect; 4 = maximal effect.
[a]Will increase dopamine activity somewhat.
Source. Adapted from Sulser F: "Pharmacology: Current Antidepressants." *Psychiatric Annals* 10:526–534, 1980; Feigner JP: "Clinical Efficacy of the Newer Antidepressants." *Journal of Clinical Psychopharmacology* 1:23S–26S, 1982; Richardson JM, Richelson E: "Antidepressants: A Clinical Update for Medical Practitioners." *Mayo Clinic Proceedings* 59:330–337, 1984; and Richelson E: "Are Receptor Studies Useful for Clinical Practice?" *Journal of Clinical Psychiatry* 44:4–9, 1983.

Table 3–4 lists these data. The information in Table 3–4 should be correlated with that in Table 3–5, which notes the signs and symptoms associated with involvement of particular sets of receptors. It then becomes easy to predict that amitriptyline is quite sedating on the basis of its strong antihistaminic effect.

Anticholinergic Effects

Anticholinergic effects are generally most evident during the first months of use. Patients will often accommodate after this. These tend to be greatest for the tertiary tricyclics (amitriptyline, imipramine, trimipramine, doxepin) and less for their demethylated metabolites. If patients are unable to tolerate them, a switch to the less anticholinergic metabolite may make sense.

Xerostomia, or *dry mouth,* can lead to stomatitis or caries. Increased fluid intake and sugarless candies or gum are often sufficient treatment. If they are not, saliva substitutes or bethanechol 10–30 mg/day divided into one or two daily doses may be added (18, 19).

Blurring for near vision secondary to mydriasis and cyclople-

---

TABLE 3–5.   **Antidepressant side effects according to receptor sites**

Anticholinergic	**Antihistamine H$_1$**
Sedation, drowsiness	Sedation
Delirium	Weight gain
Visual blurring	
Exacerbation of narrow-angle glaucoma	**α-Adrenergic blockade**
	Postural hypotension
Xerostomia (dry mouth) can lead to caries and stomatitis	Reflex tachycardia
Constipation	**Miscellaneous or unknown mechanism**
Urinary retention and hesitancy	Tremor
Sexual dysfunction	Edema
Cognitive dysfunction	
Increased heart rate	

gia also occurs. Patients should not rush to have their eyeglass prescriptions changed unless they are to stay on a stable dose for a prolonged period. Bethanechol can again be helpful, or pilocarpine 1% ophthalmic solution 1 drop qid can be administered. Patients with shallow anterior chambers are at risk for *acute narrow-angle glaucoma* if exposed to drugs that limit accommodation. Patients should be screened for this defect with the penlight test; a penlight is shone across the eye; if the nasal side of the iris fails to illuminate, the patient is at some potential risk and should have his or her intraocular pressure checked (20).

Constipation is best managed with bran, a bulk laxative, or a stool softener.

Elderly men with enlarged prostates are at particular risk for the development of *urinary retention*. If severe, there may be the need for referral to a urologist. If there is merely some urinary hesitation, bethanechol can be helpful.

The most subtle, difficult-to-diagnose toxicities are *mental status changes*. Frank delirium usually occurs when these medications are combined with other anticholinergic agents. Typically, some of the other stigmata of anticholinergic excess are evident (tachycardia, flushed facies, thirst, dry mucous membranes, enlarged pupils), but occasionally nothing is seen except mental status changes. Although most patients experience improvement in memory as the depression lifts, some elderly, cognitively compromised patients may have memory difficulties exacerbated with the addition of these agents. If a patient's memory worsens, cautious withdrawal of the antidepressant should be contemplated.

Antihistaminic Effects

Sedation is an example of a side effect that may be turned to the patient's advantage. Drugs that are potent antihistamines should be given at bedtime to assist with sleep.

Weight gain can be a problem for patients on both MAOIs and tricyclics. The mechanism is unknown, although speculation centers on an antihistaminic effect. It does not appear to simply reflect improvement of the anorexia associated with depression, because nondepressed patients with panic disorder are vulnerable to this as well. Unfortunately, there have not been good trials comparing various antidepressants, but the common practice is to switch to a less antihistaminic antidepressant if weight gain is a major problem. The SSRIs and bupropion appear to be associated with weight loss, typically insignificant, but occasionally requiring discontinuation.

Although not a toxicity, there is one further antihistaminic effect that should be noted. Both controlled and open trials support the in vitro data that trimipramine and doxepin are potent H_2 antagonists. They have compared favorably with ranitidine and cimetidine. Consequently, H_2 blockers can probably be discontinued in favor of these antidepressants (21).

α-Adrenergic Effects

Orthostatic, or postural, hypotension often impinges on antidepressant treatment, particularly in elderly, cardiovascularly compromised patients. Generally, there is more risk with tertiary tricyclics. Curiously, this liability appears to be dose related with MAOIs but not with HCAs.

Baseline orthostatic readings should always be obtained before the prescription of antidepressants. Readings should be repeated over 5–10 minutes after the patient stands. Without baseline readings, the physician is often left with the assumption that the medication is causing the postural change when other factors could be responsible. Table 3–6 lists some other common etiologies.

Patients at risk should have tertiary tricyclics or second-generation antidepressants prescribed. Symptomatic treatment may still be necessary. Restoration of fluid volume, raising the head of the bed, use of waist-high elastic support stockings, or liberalizing salt intake may be enough (22). All patients should be instructed to get up slowly from either lying or sitting. They should learn to dangle their legs over the side of the bed for several minutes before arising.

It should be remembered that it is symptoms, not numbers, that matter. Treatment should be contemplated if patients complain of lightheadedness or syncope. Many patients will be entirely asymptomatic even in the face of a 30-point drop in systolic blood pressure. Symptomatic patients who fail to respond to conservative measures may benefit from the addition of 9-α-fludrocortisone (Florinef), a mineralocorticoid that is begun at 0.1 mg/day or bid and titrated up every 5–7 days to doses as high as 1.0 mg/day. The chief risks are hypokalemia, congestive heart failure, and hypertension. All should be regularly monitored (23).

Cardiovascular Effects

The effects on blood pressure have already been reviewed. There is also an increase in heart rate, probably related to the anticholinergic effect. Since MAOIs have less anticholinergic effect, there is less associated tachycardia. Increased heart rate can be problematic for patients with unstable angina or marginally compensated congestive heart failure (24).

All HCAs with the exception of trazodone will *prolong cardiac conduction* much like quinidine, procainamide, or disopyramide. Trials have favorably compared imipramine with these type I antiarrhythmics. Patients receiving HCAs can often have their quinidine or procainamide discontinued or have the dose substantially lowered. They do carry the risk of extending any conduction

---

TABLE 3–6.   **Common causes of orthostasis**

Diabetes mellitus	Varicose veins
Parkinson's disease	Antihypertensive medication
Addison's disease	α-Adrenergic antagonists
Shy-Drager syndrome	Arrhythmia
Amyloidosis	Volume depletion: dehydration,
Prolonged bedrest	hemorrhage, etc.
Pregnancy	

abnormality. Patients with low-grade conduction abnormalities such as a first-degree atrioventricular block, a Mobitz type I second-degree atrioventricular block, a right bundle branch block, or a left anterior hemiblock should have only very cautious use of an HCA, with all dose increases accompanied by serial electrocardiograms. With these patients, bupropion, SSRIs, trazodone, an MAOI, or ECT may make more sense.

Patients with higher block (bifasicular or Mobitz type II second-degree atrioventricular blocks) should not have HCAs with the exception of trazodone, bupropion, or SSRIs under any circumstances. Trazodone has been associated with an increase in ventricular ectopy. Doxepin has been advocated by some as having less cardiovascular toxicity, but this appears to be an artifact of trials with low doses. MAOIs are remarkably well tolerated, with the exception of the associated postural hypotension. There are no data supporting any important effect of MAOIs on conduction or rhythm (24).

Miscellaneous Effects

A fine, nonparkinsonian *tremor* has been noted, especially with the more adrenergic HCAs. Discontinuation of caffeine and tobacco is frequently helpful. If symptoms persist, it may be justified to treat with a peripherally acting β-blocker.

Edema can occur. The mechanism is unknown, but has been noted in the absence of other signs of heart failure. Symptomatic treatment with low doses of a thiazide can be helpful.

Myoclonus, especially as patients are falling asleep, can occur with many antidepressants (25). This may reflect serotonergic activity and is frequently dose related. It is annoying but not dangerous. Treatment alternatives include dose reduction, change to a less serotonergic drug, or symptomatic treatment with clonazepam 0.5–1.5 mg at bedtime.

Seizures may be associated with some antidepressants. Bupropion was initially withdrawn from the market when a group of bulimic patients involved in a protocol developed a surprisingly high incidence of seizures. It was then subjected to large-scale testing before being reintroduced. It appears that it does pose a dose-related risk of seizure induction. As a result, there is a 450-mg daily maximum and a requirement that no more than 150 mg be given at one time, and the mandate that this medication not be used in patients with a history of seizure disorder or of eating disorders. Similarly heightened scrutiny with clomipramine led to a 250-mg daily maximum. The surprising aspect of this is that there are no accurate data on the likelihood of seizure generation with the older antidepressants. Although older antidepressants may pose some risk, it does not appear great (26).

Antidepressant-induced suicidality became the source of great public debate fueled by the Church of Scientology after an article appeared associating the onset of suicidal ideation with the use of fluoxetine in six quite complicated patients (27). Large-scale follow up with fluoxetine-treated patients revealed the emergence of suicidality to be a decidedly rare event (28). Review of other literature reveals that this has been reported with a wide variety of other antidepressants, and that there is a suggestion of greater antidepressant efficacy in suicidal patients with serotonergically rather than adrenergically mediated antidepressants (29). Although there is little research support for the clinical belief that suicidality can emerge when antidepressants treat the psychomotor retardation of major depression before the hopelessness, it does make sense intuitively and this stage of recovery should be a time of heightened awareness. Given the current state of knowledge, there seems little reason not to use an SSRI with a suicidally depressed patient, and the very high therapeutic index serves as an argument for such a selection.

A wide variety of *sexual difficulties* have been noted with all antidepressants, with the possible exception of bupropion. Difficulties cited include diminished libido, diminished or absent erections, ejaculatory delay or inhibition, and anorgasmia (30). Evaluation is often complicated by the residual effects of partially treated depression, which can interfere with almost all spheres of sexuality. It is extraordinarily important to ask about this area because antidepressant-induced sexual problems are quite frequent and can compromise the quality of patients' lives and their compliance. A number of alternatives can be investigated, including dose reduction, substitution of a less anticholinergic or a less serotonergically mediated antidepressant, or use of other medications as antidotes. There are no controlled studies available. Yohimbine (31), cyproheptadine, and bethanechol, typically taken several hours before sexual activity, have all been used with some success in uncontrolled trials. Trazodone has led to priapism, which can be a medical emergency. Males should be warned of this possibility and told to seek medical treatment if this side effect should occur.

Monoamine Oxidase Inhibitor Side Effects

MAOIs have minimal anticholinergic or antihistaminic effect. They are potent α-blockers and, in addition, have problems that are the direct results of inhibition of the enzyme. The predictable problems with orthostasis are the usual dose-limiting factors. Their minimal impact on muscarinic receptors, their lack of effect on cardiac conduction, and the increase in MAO activity that is seen with advanced age are making them more and more attractive to geropsychiatrists.

Monoamine Oxidase Inhibition

MAO is normally present in the gut as well as brain. One of its functions is to inactivate various pressors, notably tyramine, which is widely distributed in various foodstuffs. If these pressor agents are not inactivated, a dramatic increase in blood pressure can result. It is for this reason that patients must follow a special low-tyramine diet and must also be aware of the many potential interactions with prescribed and over-the-counter medications.

Many of the low-tyramine diets that have been published are overly restrictive, largely reflecting medical folklore rather than data. Patients often experiment with their diet, and if they experience no side effects, they go further off the diet, resulting in serious difficulty. The dietary suggestions listed in Table 3–7 include groups of foods with significant tyramine content. Patients should be instructed to completely avoid these foods.

Patients can be given photocopies of Table 3–7. It should be noted that many of the items prohibited in the past such as coffee, chocolate, and alcohol can be consumed in moderation. Patients need to carry a tyramine reference list with them and make careful inquiries in restaurants about sauces potentially containing cheese. Because MAO takes time to regenerate, patients should be instructed to start the diet 2 days before beginning an MAOI and to continue the diet for 2 weeks after discontinuation of the medication.

Drug interactions should be considered as well (Table 3–8).

TABLE 3–7.   Evidence for avoiding high-tyramine foods

Food	Case reports	Tyramine content
Aged cheeses	Many	High
Yeast extracts (usually found in health food stores; bread and other yeast products are safe)	Several	Moderate
Sauerkraut	None	High
Aged meat, sausages, cold cuts (turkey cold cuts are safe)	None	Moderate
Alcohol	Few	Low if consumed in moderation; beer should be avoided
Pickled herring	Few	Low except the brine
Liver	Few	Acceptable if fresh

Source.   Adapted from Shulman KI, Walker SE, MacKenzie S, et al: "Dietary Restriction, Tyramine, and the Use of Monoamine Oxidase Inhibitors." *Journal of Clinical Psychopharmacology* 9:397–402, 1989.

They are discussed in the section "Interactions." Many over-the-counter medications contain sympathomimetics and should be avoided. Patients should be instructed not to take any new medications until they have checked with their physician.

It is imperative that patients be properly educated about the risks of MAOIs. They are quite safe if used appropriately, but patients must be capable of understanding and following a diet or must be in a structured setting that will ensure compliance. Patients should examine the dietary restrictions before electing to receive these drugs.

Hypertensive crises fortunately are quite rare. Patients should know the symptoms associated with this reaction, including a throbbing, intense headache; flushing; nausea and vomiting; photophobia; and palpitations. Patients can be given 10 mg of nifedipine with instructions to bite the capsule and swallow the contents if symptoms occur. They should promptly seek medical attention. Significant hypertension can be treated with phentolamine 5 mg iv.

Miscellaneous Monoamine Oxidase Inhibitor Toxicities

Women may experience dose-related *anorgasmia*. Many patients find these drugs, particularly tranylcypromine, to be activating and associated with *sleep interruption*. Trazodone 25–50 mg may be used at bedtime to help with sleep. There is a remote risk of the serotonin syndrome (discussed below) with this combination, but it is generally well tolerated. Some other patients may experience severe *afternoon somnolence* when taking MAOIs (32). There is no clear-cut treatment for this side effect other than discontinuation, although some patients appear to learn how to accommodate the problem.

Paresthesia has been reported; it often responds to pyridoxine administration.

Weight gain can be a problem with many antidepressants. Tranylcypromine is the least likely of the MAOIs to have this effect (33).

TABLE 3–8. Monoamine oxidase inhibitor (MAOI) drug interactions, mechanism, and alternatives

Drug	Result and mechanism	Alternatives
Meperidine	Encephalopathy, unknown mechanism	Aspirin, acetaminophen, nonsteroidal anti-inflammatory agents, codeine, and oxycodone
Dextromethorphan	Unknown mechanism; single case report of hyperpyrexia and death; potential hypertensive crisis	Guaifenesin elixir (Robitussin), terpin hydrate with codeine
Buspirone	Increased norepinephrine	Benzodiazepines
Heterocyclic antidepressants (HCAs) and serotonin reuptake inhibitors	Fever, seizures, mechanism unknown	Two-week washout in going from an MAOI to an HCA; 1 week in going the other way; 5 weeks in going from fluoxetine to an MAOI
Sympathomimetics[a]	Hypertensive crisis	Cold, rhinitis: Antihistamines (brompheniramine, chlorpheniramine) Obesity: exercise, diet

		Anesthesia: for local, use non-epinephrine-containing lidocaine or procaine; for major surgery, washout 2 weeks in advance; in an emergency, correct hypotension with fluids; avoid succinylcholine
Succinylcholine	Prolonged muscle relaxation	See above
Electroconvulsive therapy	Potential hypertension because of increased catecholamines	Washout 2 weeks before
Methyldopa Clonidine High-dose β-blockers Guanethidine Reserpine	Hypotension	Diuretics Vasodilators Angiotensin-converting enzyme inhibitors

[a] Amphetamine, L-dopa, ephedrine, epinephrine, isoproterenol, metaraminol, methylphenidate, norepinephrine, phenylephrine, phenylpropanolamine, pseudoephedrine, and others.

Management of Overdose

Traditional Heterocyclics

HCAs are the leading cause of death from intentional overdose. This unfortunate statistic reflects both how dangerous they can be and how much the population taking them is at risk. The primary difficulties are cardiac, but seizures and anticholinergic effects can complicate the situation greatly. Most difficulties occur within the first 6 hours, but the anticholinergic effects can occur later because of marked delays in absorption. The majority of deaths are because of cardiac difficulties and occur within the first 24 hours. They are usually associated with doses in excess of 1,250 mg of imipramine or equivalent. This is the basis for prescribing only 1 week's medication at a time if there is concern about a patient's suicidality.

Fortunately, difficulties do not occur once the patient has regained alertness and the electrocardiogram has normalized. The electrocardiogram is quite predictive of toxicity. If the maximal QRS duration is less than 100 milliseconds, the risk of arrhythmia and of seizures is negligible. If the QRS is between 100 and 160 milliseconds, there is a moderate risk for seizures, but little for arrhythmia; if it is greater than 160 milliseconds, the risk is high for both (34). A wide variety of arrhythmias are seen. Patients may become hypotensive as a function of α-blockade. All overdoses with HCAs should be taken seriously and treated aggressively.

Second-Generation Heterocyclics

Amoxapine, maprotiline, and bupropion all carry the primary risk of seizures with overdose but appear to be relatively well tolerated in terms of cardiac toxicity. Fluoxetine seems relatively benign. There are few data available about sertraline or paroxetine.

Monoamine Oxidase Inhibitors

Toxicity is usually manifested by central nervous system hyperactivity with agitation, hyperreflexia, and rigidity. Both hyper- and hypotension have been reported. Death, coma, and arrhythmia are all rare.

■ WITHDRAWAL OF ANTIDEPRESSANTS

Heterocyclics

Abrupt discontinuation of an antidepressant can be associated either with development of a withdrawal syndrome or with reemergence of the depression. Therefore, medications should be gradually tapered in an attempt to establish whether there is a lower, effective dose. Withdrawal effects can include anxiety, restlessness, diarrhea, a flulike syndrome, piloerection, and, rarely, delirium and mania (35).

Monoamine Oxidase Inhibitors

Evidence of a withdrawal syndrome is lacking, although reemergent depression may occur with MAOIs just as with HCAs. It must be remembered that it will take 2 weeks for MAO to regenerate. Patients must maintain their diets and be wary of interactions for this period.

■ INTERACTIONS

Monoamine Oxidase Inhibitor and Heterocyclic Use

For populations of patients, there are no data indicating that coprescription of MAOIs and HCAs is any better than using either drug alone. It is clear, however, that individual patients refractory to both drugs can respond to the combination. If precautions are not taken this can be a very dangerous combination, resulting in hyperpyrexia, convulsions, tremor, increased tone, and coma. If guidelines are followed, the combination can be managed safely (36). *HCAs should never be added to an MAOI without an intervening 2-week washout.* Ideally, there should be a medication-free period followed by concurrent initiation of the antidepressants. The preferred HCAs are amitriptyline, doxepin, and trimipramine. Imipramine and desipramine should not be used. Phenelzine should be chosen over tranylcypromine. Doses should be gradually increased. The final doses are dependent on the outcome, but full antidepressant regimens of both are frequently required. This approach is best reserved for the patient who fails to respond to more conventional regimens.

Heterocyclics

HCAs are metabolized via the cytochrome P-450 system. Other drugs that are metabolized in this way (phenothiazines, alcohol, cimetidine, disulfiram, oral contraceptives) will result in increased levels of themselves and of the tricyclic if coadministered. Smoking and barbiturates induce the same system and result in lower HCA levels. This is not problematic if the doses of all drugs remain constant, because levels would then remain constant. Plasma levels are higher for blacks than for whites and are increased by weight loss (12). Fluoxetine is a potent inhibitor of the P-450 system and can lead to significant increases in plasma levels of many tricyclics. This is particularly problematic given the long half-life of norfluoxetine (37). Sertraline has little impact on the P-450 system, paroxetine a bit more.

HCAs act by blocking reuptake into the presynaptic neuron. This means that antihypertensives such as guanethidine are ineffective. Sympathomimetics, on the other hand, have a greatly augmented effect, to the point where hypertensive crisis may eventuate. This is because their effect is not terminated by reuptake as is usually the case.

A serotonin syndrome has been reported, most typically with the addition of L-tryptophan (a serotonergic precursor currently withdrawn from the United States market because of an eosinophilia-myalgia syndrome) to fluoxetine or an MAOI. The syndrome is typically characterized by mental status changes, restlessness, myoclonus, hyperreflexia, diaphoresis, shivering, and tremor. Treatment consists of discontinuing the offending serotonergic agents and supportive care. The bulk of the difficulty should resolve within a day, but confusion may linger for several days (38). Similar difficulties have been noted when pro-serotonergic agents have been combined.

Additive effects are predictable with other agents that are anticholinergic or α-blockers.

Although lithium is generally well tolerated when combined with fluoxetine, there are case reports of neurotoxicity. This is a sufficiently rare occurrence so as not to preclude coadministration.

■ AN APPROACH TO THE DEPRESSED PATIENT

A wide variety of treatments are available for people with depression. Some are more effective than others for particular sub-populations of depressed patients. Moreover, every clinician cannot be equally facile with all of the available treatment options; instead it makes sense to become well acquainted with several of the available alternatives. With this background it becomes clear that there cannot be a broad consensus supporting any particular treatment approach. Each clinician should, however, develop a sequence of treatment options that he or she is comfortable with. The therapies should follow each other logically. The long-range plan should be thought out so that the clinician anticipates what steps would follow if a particular therapeutic approach fails.

What follows is but one series of options. There are considerable grounds for disagreement; many would prefer to try several HCAs before moving on to an MAOI or ECT. This is a perfectly defensible point of view. Rather than suggesting that this is the only appropriate treatment course, the aim is to suggest that a series of logical options should be entertained from the beginning.

Before beginning, several assumptions about the patient need to be clarified. The first is that the correct diagnosis is depression. A structured interview is helpful. At a minimum, DSM-IV should be used (2). Diagnosis of melancholia by these criteria is encouraging as a predictor of response. Use of the Hamilton Depression Rating Scale is also helpful (39).

In addition to establishing the diagnosis, thorough physical and laboratory examinations must be done to rule out organic etiologies for the depression and to ensure that the patient can tolerate medication safely. A careful history should be taken with special attention paid to understanding the patient's previous response to medication. Always begin with whichever medication previously worked. If there is no previous antidepressant use, inquiries should be made about other family members' responses. In the absence of other data, it is prudent to begin with whatever has been helpful for relatives with similar illnesses.

Selection of an Initial Treatment

Ordinarily, treatment should begin with an HCA. Exceptions include

1. Past history of response to ECT or an MAOI
2. An atypical depression with hyperphagia, hypersomnolence, a sense of leaden paralysis, anxiety, and emotional hyperactivity
3. Cardiac conduction defects that would suggest use of an SSRI, bupropion, trazodone, an MAOI, or ECT

If there is no contraindication, use nortriptyline, imipramine, or desipramine because plasma levels are best delineated for these drugs. Nortriptyline is significantly more expensive than imipramine or desipramine.

Treatment would ordinarily begin with 50 mg of imipramine or desipramine or 25 mg of nortriptyline given at bedtime. If tolerated well, the dose should be increased by a like amount every 3 days until the patient is taking 200 mg of imipramine or desipramine or 100 mg of nortriptyline at bedtime. If after 3 weeks there is an insufficient response, a plasma level should be checked with a reliable laboratory and the dose appropriately titrated. If the patient responds positively, and if this was a relatively benign first episode, then the medicine should be maintained for 16–20 weeks after maximal relief is obtained. If the patient has a recurrent depressive illness, treatment should probably continue for years.

Augmentation Strategies

The nonresponsive patient might benefit from the addition of lithium or triiodothyronine. The addition of lithium to both HCAs and MAOIs has been helpful for many treatment-refractory patients. Initial investigation was spurred by the fact that lithium serves to increase levels of serotonin. Its role in augmentation seems independent of its function as a thymoleptic because the response is often evident within a week and low doses (e.g., 300 mg tid) generally prove helpful. Similar results were obtained for both HCAs and MAOIs (40, 41), and in patients with both bipolar and unipolar depression (42). There have been conflicting data on the use of triiodothyronine, but a recent well-controlled trial found both lithium and 37.5 µg/day of liothyronine to be superior to placebo in the treatment of tricyclic-nonresponsive depressed patients (43).

There is considerable reliance on lithium augmentation in this approach. This is because of both its efficacy and the rapidity of response. No more than a week is lost by such an intervention. Although recent data indicate that the full response may well take 3 weeks or more, some measure of improvement is usually apparent more rapidly (42). A positive response should lead to maintenance for the same period, described previously.

Second-Level Treatments

If a patient fails to respond to these initial treatments, several options can be considered. An MAOI, another HCA, a second-generation antidepressant, or ECT could all be appropriate. An MAOI has a reasonably high likelihood of benefit, but significantly limits the available options if it fails (44, 45). A good trial of an MAOI takes over a month followed by a 2-week washout before other treatments can be considered. One HCA may work after another fails, but the likelihood of response is somewhat less than for the other options. A second-generation antidepressant would mean another class of medication that seems logical.

If an MAOI is chosen and the patient fails to respond to 3 weeks of 1 mg/kg body weight of phenelzine or 0.5 mg/kg body weight of tranylcypromine, lithium augmentation should be used as previously described. If this fails, a 2-week washout should be followed by ECT. Patients responding to an MAOI should be maintained on medication as previously described.

The small percentage of patients who are nonresponsive to ECT should probably provoke diagnostic reexamination. If such a search confirms the diagnosis of major depression, a trial of an MAOI should be considered if not previously attempted. ECT is discussed in detail in Chapter 5.

The Treatment-Refractory Patient

A depressed patient who fails to respond to the previously discussed regimens might be considered truly treatment refractory. A series of alternatives for these patients follows. Each treatment is of relatively low yield for populations of patients, but some individuals do respond. Therefore, a continued search may well be justified (46).

Lithium or Carbamazepine Alone

Lithium and carbamazepine both are rather indifferent antidepressants, although they have great value in preventing the return of unipolar depression. Despite the lack of statistical efficacy in treating populations of depressed patients, they do have a clear value for some individuals. They should, however, be consigned to the bottom of the list with other relatively low-yield procedures (47). When added to carbamazepine, lithium appears to effectively convert a significant number of previously unresponsive patients with bipolar depression (48).

Stimulants

Despite widespread use for depression after their development in the 1930s, there has been remarkably little systematic research on stimulants (49). Their use has been advocated, especially in medically ill patients intolerant of more conventional antidepressant treatment (50). They are generally well tolerated and are particularly helpful for psychomotorically retarded, apathetic, withdrawn patients. It is less clear whether the effect lasts beyond several weeks because the few trials in the literature report only on short-term use. The risks include precipitation of a paranoid psychosis, tolerance, insomnia, and anorexia, as well as rebound depression and fatigue with discontinuation of the drug. Trials may nonetheless be warranted in depressed patients unresponsive to more orthodox therapies. The response is usually rapid, so benefit should be apparent within 2 weeks. The most commonly used agents are dextroamphetamine sulfate 10–30 mg/day and methylphenidate 10–40 mg/day. Doses should be split and given in the morning to avoid the insomnia associated with their use. The potential for habituation and the lack of controlled support for their use in depression leave them reserved for the treatment-refractory or medically compromised patient intolerant of more usual antidepressants (51).

Sleep Deprivation

A significant percentage of patients with major depression will respond positively to a night of sleep deprivation. This is especially true for those patients with diurnal variation worse in the morning. Waking patients at 2 A.M. and keeping them awake throughout the next day is as effective as a full night without sleep for most patients who respond to treatment. Unfortunately, the overwhelming majority will relapse rapidly when they are allowed to return to uninterrupted sleep. Some patients have maintained the initial response if they were placed on lithium or clomipramine concurrent with the sleep deprivation. It should be noted that studies have not been done with truly treatment-refractory patients. There is also an indication that sleep deprivation might be a way of distinguishing between dementia and depressive pseudodementia because the latter group is far more likely to have a positive response to sleep deprivation (52).

■ REFERENCES

1. DiMascio A, Weissman MM, Prosoff BA, et al: Differential symptom reduction by drugs and psychotherapy in acute depression. Arch Gen Psychiatry 36:1450–1456, 1979
2. American Psychiatric Association: Diagnostic and Statistical Manual of Mental Disorders, 4th Edition. Washington, DC, American Psychiatric Association, 1994
3. Prien RF, Kupfer DJ: Continuation drug therapy for major depressive episodes: how long should it be maintained? Am J Psychiatry 143:18–23, 1986
4. Kupfer DJ, Frank E, Perel JM, et al: Five-year outcome for maintenance therapies in recurrent depression. Arch Gen Psychiatry 49:769–773, 1992
5. Spiker DG, Weiss JC, Dealy RS, et al: The pharmacological treatment of delusional depression. Am J Psychiatry 142:430–436, 1985
6. Keller MB, Lavori PW, Rice J, et al: The persistent risk of chronicity in recurrent episodes of nonbipolar major depressive disorder: a prospective follow-up. Am J Psychiatry 143:224–228, 1986
7. Howland RH: Pharmacotherapy of dysthymia: a review. J Clin Psychopharmacol 11:83–92, 1991
8. McGrath PJ, Stewart JW, Harrison WM, et al: Predictive value of symptoms of atypical depression for differential drug treatment outcome. J Clin Psychopharmacol 12:197–202, 1992

9. Stewart JW, McGrath PJ, Quitkin FM: Can mildly depressed outpatients with atypical depression benefit from antidepressants? Am J Psychiatry 149:615–619, 1992

10. Blehar MC, Lewy AJ: Seasonal mood disorders: consensus and controversy. Psychopharmacol Bull 26:465–494, 1990

11. American Psychiatric Association: Tricyclic antidepressants—blood level measurements and clinical outcome: an APA task force report. Am J Psychiatry 142:155–162, 1985

12. Charney DS, Menkes DB, Heninger GB: Receptor sensitivity and the mechanism of action of antidepressant treatment. Arch Gen Psychiatry 38:1160–1180, 1981

13. Rizack MA, Hillman CDM (eds): The Medical Letter Handbook of Adverse Drug Interactions. New Rochelle, NY, The Medical Letter, 1985

14. Amin M, Lehmann H, Mirmiran J: A double-blind, placebo-controlled dose-finding study with sertraline. Psychopharmacol Bull 25:164–167, 1989

15. Wilens TE, Biederman J, Baldessarini RJ, et al: Fluoxetine inhibits desipramine metabolism (letter). Arch Gen Psychiatry 49:752, 1992

16. Consensus Development Panel: Mood disorders: pharmacologic prevention of recurrences. Am J Psychiatry 142:469–476, 1985

17. Frank E, Kupfer DJ, Perel JM, et al: Three-year outcomes for maintenance therapies in recurrent depression. Arch Gen Psychiatry 47:1093–1099, 1990

18. Pollack MH, Rosenbaum JF: Management of antidepressant-induced side effects: a practical guide for the clinician. J Clin Psychiatry 48:3–8, 1987

19. Treatment of xerostomia. The Medical Letter 30:74–76, 1988

20. Lieberman E, Stoudemire A: Use of tricyclic antidepressants in patients with glaucoma. Psychosomatics 28:145–148, 1987

21. Haggerty JJ, Brossman DA: Psychotropic drugs: use in peptic ulcer patients. Psychosomatics 26:277–284, 1985

22. Ornot J, Golberg MR, Hollister AS, et al: Management of chronic orthostatic hypotension. Am J Med 80:454–464, 1986

23. Schatz IJ: Current management concepts in orthostatic hypotension. Arch Intern Med 140:1152–1154, 1980
24. Goldstein MG, Guttmacher LB: Treatment of the cardiac-impaired depressed patient, part I: general considerations, heterocyclic antidepressants, and monoamine oxidase inhibitors. Psychiatr Med 6:1–33, 1988
25. Garvey M, Tollefson G: Occurrence of myoclonus in patients treated with cyclic antidepressants. Arch Gen Psychiatry 44:269–272, 1987
26. Jick SS, Jick H, Knauss TA, et al: Antidepressants and convulsions. J Clin Psychopharmacol 12:241–245, 1992
27. Teicher MH, Glod C, Cole JO: Emergence of intense suicidal preoccupation during fluoxetine treatment. Am J Psychiatry 147:207–210, 1990
28. Beasley CM, Dornseif BE, Bosomworth JC, et al: Fluoxetine and suicide: a meta-analysis of controlled trials of treatment for depression. BMJ 303:685–692, 1991
29. Mann JJ, Kapur S: The emergence of suicidal ideation and behavior during antidepressant pharmacotherapy. Arch Gen Psychiatry 48:1027–1033, 1991
30. Segraves RT: Sexual dysfunction complicating the treatment of depression. J Clin Psychiatry Monograph 10(1):75–79, 1992
31. Hollander E, McCarley A: Yohimbine treatment of sexual side effects induced by serotonin reuptake blockers. J Clin Psychiatry 53:207–209, 1992
32. Teicher MH, Cohen BM, Baldessarini RJ, et al: Severe daytime somnolence in patients treated with an MAOI. Am J Psychiatry 145:1552–1556, 1988
33. Cantu TG, Korek JS: Monoamine oxidase inhibitors and weight gain. Drug Intelligence and Clinical Pharmacology 22:755–759, 1988
34. Boehnert MT, Lovejoy FH: Value of the QRS duration versus the serum drug level in predicting seizures and ventricular arrhythmias after an acute overdose of tricyclic antidepressants. N Engl J Med 313:474–479, 1985

35. Dilsalver SC, Greden JF: Antidepressant withdrawal phenomena. Biol Psychiatry 19:237–256, 1984

36. White K, Simpson G: Combined MAOI–tricyclic antidepressant treatment: a reevaluation. J Clin Psychopharmacol 1:264–282, 1981

37. Ciraulo DA, Shader RI: Fluoxetine drug-drug interactions, I: antidepressants and antipsychotics. J Clin Psychopharmacol 10:48–50, 1990

38. Sternbach H: The serotonin syndrome. Am J Psychiatry 148:705–713, 1991

39. Williams JBW: A structured interview guide for the Hamilton Depression Rating Scale. Arch Gen Psychiatry 45:742–747, 1988

40. DeMontigny C, Cournoyer G, Morrissette R, et al: Lithium carbonate addition in tricyclic antidepressant–resistant unipolar depression. Arch Gen Psychiatry 40:1327–1334, 1983

41. Price LH, Charney DS, Heninger GR: Efficacy of lithium-tranylcypromine treatment in refractory depression. Am J Psychiatry 142:619–623, 1985

42. Price LH, Charney DS, Heninger GR: Variability of response to lithium augmentation in refractory depression. Am J Psychiatry 143:1387–1392, 1986

43. Joffe RT, Singer W, Levitt AJ: A placebo-controlled comparison of lithium and triiodothyronine augmentation of tricyclic antidepressants in unipolar refractory depression. Arch Gen Psychiatry 50:387–393, 1993

44. McGrath PJ, Stewart JW, Harrison W, et al: Treatment of tricyclic refractory depression with a monoamine oxidase inhibitor. Psychopharmacol Bull 23:169–172, 1987

45. Thase ME, Mullinger AG, McKnight D, et al: Treatment of imipramine-resistant recurrent depression, IV: a double-blind study of tranylcypromine for anergic bipolar depression. Am J Psychiatry 149:195–198, 1992

46. Nierenberg AA, White K: What next? a review of pharmacologic strategies for treatment resistant depression. Psychopharmacol Bull 26:429–460, 1990

47. Post RM, Uhde TW, Roy-Byrne PP, et al: Antidepressant effects of carbamazepine. Am J Psychiatry 143:29–34, 1986

48. Kramlinger KG, Post RM: The addition of lithium to carbamazepine: antidepressant efficacy in treatment-resistant depression. Arch Gen Psychiatry 46:794–800, 1989

49. Chiarello RJ, Cole JO: The use of psychostimulants in general psychiatry. Arch Gen Psychiatry 44:286–295, 1987

50. Kaufmann MW, Murray GB, Cassem NH: Use of psychostimulants in medically ill depressed patients. Psychosomatics 23:817–819, 1982

51. Satel SL, Nelson JC: Stimulants in the treatment of depression: a critical overview. J Clin Psychiatry 50:241–249, 1989

52. Leibenluft E, Wehr TA: Is sleep deprivation useful in the treatment of depression? Am J Psychiatry 149:159–168, 1992

AGENTS FOR BIPOLAR DISORDER

■ HISTORY

Lithium was widely used in patent medicines and as a salt substitute for almost a century. In 1949, Cade, working in a remote Australian laboratory, reported on 19 psychiatric patients who received lithium. Even with this limited sample, he was able to note an antimanic effect but saw little impact on schizophrenic or on acutely depressed patients (1). It was 20 years before lithium was fully approved in the United States. It is now the cornerstone of treatment for acute mania and for prophylaxis with patients with unipolar and bipolar diseases. Recently, alternative agents have been investigated. Carbamazepine, marketed as an anticonvulsant, is known to have a similar therapeutic profile but different toxicities. Valproate is emerging as yet another alternative. Other anticonvulsants and calcium channel blockers are in the early stages of investigation.

■ LITHIUM

Indications

Mania

Lithium is clearly superior to placebo in acute mania. There is more of a question surrounding its role vis á vis antipsychotics, which are also helpful. Lithium's onset is slower, often not being fully apparent until 5–10 days after therapeutic levels are obtained (2). Antipsychotics work more quickly and are preferred when rapid behavioral control is necessary. Lithium has the advantage of creating less sedation. Those patients who are to be maintained on lithium can have it added, with the antipsychotic weaned once therapeutic lithium levels are obtained. The usual "therapeutic" blood level is between 0.8 and 1.5 mmol/L. This range is based on large populations of patients. Any individual can be outside these limits and still do quite well.

Not all patients with mania should receive thymoleptics. Maintenance treatment would not be justified for patients who cycle very infrequently because the potential for toxicity would outweigh the potential gain. An acute episode can often be managed with antipsychotics, unless thymoleptics are to be used for maintenance. Patients with repeated seasonal illnesses may be able to manage by taking medication only at the time of year when they are vulnerable. Deciding on which patients with recurrent illnesses should be treated requires considerable wisdom. Table 4–1 summarizes some of the points that should be considered. This decision should be discussed in a forthright fashion with the patient and his or her family.

Depression

There are conflicting data about lithium's role in the acute treatment of depression, although it is clearly not a first-line treatment

---

TABLE 4–1. **Arguments for and against pharmacologic treatment of recurrent illness**

Arguments for treatment	**Arguments against treatment**
Sudden deterioration without promontory warnings or insights	Good relationships between the physician, patient, and patient's family so that exacerbations will be reported early
Marked behavioral dyscontrol with negative consequences	
Strong family history	Prominent early warning signs such as decreased sleep or increased energy
Absence of medication toxicity	
Frequent cycling	Illnesses that respond rapidly to treatment
	Infrequent cycling
	Exacerbations that do not include serious consequences
	Toxic medications

(3). The stronger the patient's or patient's family history of bipolar disease, the more likely the patient is to respond to lithium when he or she is depressed. Support for lithium augmentation of antidepressants is clearer. There are suggestions that heterocyclic antidepressants (HCAs) may accelerate cycling in patients with bipolar disease (4). Lithium does not share this liability.

Prevention of Recurrent Affective Disorders

It is in this area that lithium's effects are most dramatic. Lithium will decrease the number and severity of manic episodes and the number of depressive episodes. The intermorbid interval will be extended as well. Even if patients are fully compliant, symptoms may break through; lithium's prevention is relative, not absolute.

The extent to which lithium levels should be lowered for maintenance has been the subject of considerable debate. In a recent study patients were randomly assigned to groups that received lithium at levels of either 0.4–0.6 mmol/L or 0.8–1.0 mmol/L (5). The group with the lower level had a 2.6-fold increase in their rate of relapse. Side effects, most noticeably tremor, diarrhea, increased urinary frequency, weight gain, and a metallic taste, were higher in the high-dose group. Based on this study, the best suggestion would be to aim for the higher dose and see if the patient is able to tolerate it. If side effects become significant, the choice becomes either the low-dose approach or switching to an alternative agent.

Predictors of the likelihood of patients responding to lithium prophylactically are beginning to emerge. Those patients with a family history of bipolar disorder, good intermorbid functioning, increased likelihood of compliance, and depressive episodes following mania are more likely to respond. Poor prognostic signs include mixed episodes with both depressive and manic features coexisting, substance abuse, having four or more episodes annually, and cycling from depression into mania (6). None of these predictors are absolute, and they should not preclude the prophylactic use of lithium. Negative prognostic features should cause the clinician to consider anticonvulsants more seriously.

In patients with unipolar disease there is equally strong support for the use of either lithium or antidepressants (7). The choice should be based on which agent is most likely to enhance compliance, although in the presence of a strong family history of bipolar disorder there would be some argument for lithium instead of an antidepressant.

Schizophrenia, Schizoaffective Disorder

Approximately one-half of correctly diagnosed schizophrenic patients will show some improvement if lithium is added to their antipsychotic. The response rate is even higher if there is a strong affective component to the illness (8). Affective symptoms are most likely to respond but there can be some improvement in core schizophrenic symptoms such as hallucinations, delusions, and formal thought disorder as well (9). Overall the response is less robust than in affective disorder but is sufficient to justify a trial, usually by adding lithium to antipsychotics, in treatment-refractory patients.

Alcoholism

A recent trial followed alcoholic patients for 1 year undergoing conventional alcohol treatment combined with lithium or a placebo; lithium enhanced the chance of sobriety in compliant patients. This is discussed in more detail in Chapter 8.

Aggression

Lithium, when administered to prisoners lacking any psychiatric diagnosis, led to a significant decrease in episodes of aggression when compared with a placebo. Case reports also support its use in controlling aggressive outbursts in developmentally disabled and dementia patients, but there are no controlled studies. The use of lithium, carbamazepine, and β-blockers all have preliminary support, but there is no definitive treatment. This is discussed in Chapter 8.

Toxicities

Most patients on lithium have some sort of toxic effects. Generally, they are quite mild and well tolerated (10).

Intoxication

Levels are a good guide to dosage, but should always be tempered with a physical examination. The signs of lithium intoxication are predictable and dose related (11). Considerable effort should be expended in educating patients about the signs and symptoms associated with toxicity so that they can obtain help promptly. Table 4–2 includes the levels usually associated with particular toxicities.

A fine *tremor* is frequent, even at therapeutic doses. It rarely interferes with function, but some patients, such as musicians or surgeons, find it problematic. In these cases waiting for accommodation, reduction of dose, decreasing caffeine consumption, or low doses of a β-blocker are all valid alternatives.

Lithium is a gastric irritant and should not be taken on an empty stomach. Even eating a few crackers before taking the medicine will be helpful; it should normally be given after meals. If nausea does eventuate, switching to an extended-release preparation is the best alternative.

There should not be exclusive reliance on the plasma level as

TABLE 4–2.   **Lithium levels and toxicity**

- **Early and benign**
  Tremor, nausea, polydipsia, polyuria
- **Levels at or above 1.5 mmol/L**
  Diarrhea, vomiting, drowsiness, weakness, and decreased coordination
- **Levels above 2.5 mmol/L**
  Ataxia, dizziness, tinnitus, blurred vision, cogwheeling, dysphasia, delirium, muscle twitching, hyperreflexia, fasciculations, focal neurological signs, seizures, hyperpyrexia, coma

a measure of lithium toxicity after an overdose because it may be a poor reflection of what is going on in the brain. *Delirium* has persisted for days or weeks following peripheral normalization (12). Severe overdoses are managed with dialysis. More moderate cases are treated by osmotic diuresis, vigorous hydration, and alkalinized urine.

Endocrine

Hypothyroidism, by either laboratory or clinical parameters, occurs in 5%–15% of long-term lithium patients. It is far more common in women and often occurs during the first 6 months of therapy (13). This is not necessarily an indication to discontinue lithium, and many patients are managed effectively with thyroid replacement. Because many of the symptoms of hypothyroidism mimic those of depression, it is always wise to check the thyroid function of a previously stable lithium patient who becomes depressed. More rarely, patients develop hyperthyroidism. *Thyroid abnormality* is more common in patients with previous history or family history of thyroid difficulties. Consequently it is wise to obtain baseline triiodothyronine, thyroxine, and thyroid-stimulating hormone (TSH) assays. TSH should probably be monitored on a semiannual basis thereafter or whenever there is clinical suspicion of abnormality. Thyroid dysfunction should reverse with discontinuation of lithium.

Patients taking lithium long term may develop statistically significant increases in calcium, ionized calcium, and parathyroid hormone levels (14). Although it is decidedly unusual for this to be clinically evident, patients who develop ataxia, weakness, confusion, depression, and lethargy while taking lithium should have a calcium level determination done. Parathyroid hyperplasia may occur with long-term use (15).

It is quite common to gain weight while taking lithium. Multiple factors are probably involved. Lithium has a similar effect to insulin on carbohydrate metabolism. Patients may develop polydipsia and look to high-calorie liquids to quench their thirst. They are often coprescribed antidepressants and antipsychotics, which are also associated with *weight gain*. Patients, particularly those with a history of obesity, should be forewarned about this possibility and urged to exercise dietary caution.

Renal and Electrolyte

Lithium is primarily excreted through the kidneys. It is reabsorbed in the proximal tubule with sodium and water, but unlike sodium there is no further excretion in the distal nephron. If the body is experiencing a relative sodium deficiency it compensates by reabsorbing more sodium than normal proximally; lithium is absorbed with it. Hence, the risk of lithium toxicity follows hyponatremia. Patients should be instructed to increase their salt intake in the event of exercise, fever, or other sources of increased diaphoresis. Sodium-wasting diuretics can be used with caution, but it should be realized that there will be an attendant increase in lithium levels.

It has long been noted that manic patients seem to require more lithium to achieve a specific level. There is a suspicion that lithium clearance may be state dependent, but this has not been documented.

For many patients, lithium diminishes the response of adenylate cyclase to vasopressin and therefore the ability to concentrate their urine. This is termed *nephrogenic diabetes insipidus* (NDI). NDI is related to cumulative lithium exposure. The result is that patients put out large quantities of dilute urine. This condition generally reverses after discontinuation of the drug. Significant polyuria is difficult for many patients to tolerate. If suspected, the clinician should monitor urine osmolality and 24-hour urine volume. If tests indicate the presence of NDI, the alternatives are to discontinue lithium or to administer amiloride 5 mg bid along with the lithium (16).

Rarely, lithium patients present with the nephrotic syndrome secondary to glomerular nephritis. This typically reverses with discontinuation of the lithium. Whether lithium causes diminution in the *glomerular filtration rate* (GFR) is less clear. Good studies require the use of a control group of patients with affective disorder who are not on lithium to ascertain if the drug itself is causing the change. It seems likely that there is a statistical, but small, decrease in the GFR with long-term lithium use, but significant decreases are rare (17). The decrease in the GFR is presumably secondary to tubulointerstitial nephropathy (18). There is a suspicion that these effects relate to cumulative exposure and therefore it would be prudent to maintain the lowest effective level of lithium. Serum creatinine and urine should be monitored at baseline and every 4–6 months for patients on maintenance. If there is any evidence of proteinuria or of a rising creatinine level, more elaborate testing of renal functioning should be performed.

Edema is occasionally noted in patients on lithium. It is typically mild, transient, and localized to the pretibial area. It is not usually sufficient to warrant treatment, but does respond to diuretics, which should be used cautiously because of the risk of inducing lithium intoxication (19).

Cardiovascular

One-quarter of patients on lithium will develop reversible, nonspecific *T wave changes* similar to those seen with hypokalemia. Lithium replaces intracellular potassium; thus, the T wave changes may reflect decreased intracellular potassium stores, although serum potassium remains within normal limits. *Sinus node dysfunction* has been reported, but other arrhythmias are rare (20).

Dermatologic

Psoriatic and *acneiform lesions* have been reported as well as various rashes. Caution should be exercised in patients with preexistent psoriasis because lithium can lead to significant exacerbation. Lithium use can also lead to hair loss.

Hematopoietic

Lithium induces a reversible *leukocytosis* that remains so long as the drug is maintained. White blood cell counts of 13,000–

15,000/mm^3 are not unusual. The increase is usually in granulo-cytes and represents a step-up in the total-body white blood cell count, rather than margination. The effect is so predictable that lithium is being used as an adjunct to some chemotherapeutic programs. There are no other known hematologic effects.

Neurological

Many of the signs and symptoms discussed in the section about intoxication are neurological. Occasionally, patients develop *par-kinsonian symptoms* when taking therapeutic doses of lithium. Cogwheeling is usually the most prominent symptom. It appears less responsive than neuroleptic-induced extrapyramidal syn-dromes to antiparkinsonian agents. There may be a subtle motor slowing, but there is no evidence for any cognitive effect secondary to the medication (21). There is continued debate about the effect of lithium on creativity. For a minority of patients, episodes of hypomania may well be connected with enhanced creativity. Such patients would associate lithium and euthymia with dulled creativ-ity; for most patients, productivity is enhanced.

Pharmacology

Lithium is a simple salt. There are several preparations available. Standard lithium carbonate is rapidly absorbed with peak blood levels obtained after about 2 hours. The elimination half-life for a single dose is about 8 hours and in the 18- to 36-hour range when steady state is obtained. It differs from most psychotropics because it is not protein bound, does not have any metabolites, and is trapped in several organs including the kidney and thyroid. It is almost entirely excreted through the kidneys, with minor amounts in saliva, sweat, tears, and semen. Lithium levels could be moni-tored in any of these fluids, but custom dictates blood plasma levels with blood drawn approximately 12 hours after the last dose.

There are three different lithium preparations available in the United States: conventional lithium carbonate, available in 300-

and 450-mg tablets and capsules; lithium citrate, a liquid with 5 ml being equivalent to 300 mg; and extended-release lithium carbonate preparations.

Lithium citrate is used in patients who cannot swallow pills or are at high risk for hiding pills in their mouth and not swallowing them and in geriatric patients where adjustment of the dose requires increments of less than 300 mg. Extended-release preparations are indicated when there is gastrointestinal toxicity or where twice-daily dosing would enhance compliance. They are, however, more expensive.

Lithium is usually given either three or four times per day. Some advocate once-daily dosing with an extended-release preparation based on the belief that the peak after absorption offers psychiatric protection and the lower levels that would follow throughout the rest of the day would offer some protection to the kidney. There are not sufficient data at this point to justify this, but it is clear that many patients can do well with such a regimen. The major problem is gastric irritation with one large daily dose. If such a regimen is used, it should be realized that the 12-hour trough level will be higher than that for the same total daily dose taken more frequently.

Conventional lithium carbonate is usually begun at a dose of 300 mg tid for a normal-size patient, then titrated by physical examination and blood levels to a target level. Dose adjustments and levels can be done every 3–5 days.

Lithium discontinuation, even if done abruptly, is not associated with physical problems. The chief difficulty is the possibility of relapse. If lithium is to be discontinued, it should be done over the course of several weeks, because rapid discontinuation is associated with increased risk of relapse (22).

Laboratory Monitoring

Table 4–3 contains one set of recommendations for routine monitoring of lithium. After the dose is stabilized, the level will remain relatively constant, barring a change in the patient's physical or mental status. Until the medication regimen has stabilized, levels will need to be drawn more frequently. Any elevation in the creatinine blood level should be followed with a 24-hour creatinine clearance corrected for age and surface area.

Interactions

Table 4–4 lists some of the more frequently reported interactions (23). At one time there was great concern about interactions with haloperidol. In retrospect, the reports may be variants of neuroleptic malignant syndrome, and haloperidol may have been implicated simply because it is a commonly prescribed high-potency agent. The reaction is sufficiently rare that coprescription is quite justified, but an alert eye should be maintained. Because of the prolongation of the succinylcholine's effect, lithium should be discontinued for 48 hours before electroconvulsive therapy (ECT).

■ CARBAMAZEPINE

Carbamazepine is a tricyclic anticonvulsant commonly used for the treatment of complex partial and tonic-clonic seizures. It is

---

TABLE 4–3.   **Routine laboratory monitoring of lithium**

- **At baseline**
  Triiodothyronine (T_3), thyroxine (T_4), thyroid-stimulating hormone
  Serum creatinine
  Urinalysis
  Electrocardiogram, if cardiac risk factors exist
- **Every 6 months**
  Serum creatinine
  Urinalysis
  Thyroid-stimulating hormone
- **Lithium levels, once stable, can be checked every 3 months**

TABLE 4–4. **Lithium drug interactions**

Drug	Effect
ACE inhibitors	Lithium levels increase.
Antipsychotics	Coprescription, especially with high-potency agents, may increase the risk of neuroleptic malignant syndrome, although it is not clear if this is because of affective disorder or lithium. Somnambulism has also been reported.
Benzodiazepines	Long-term coprescription may cause increased sexual dysfunction.[a]
Carbamazepine	Occasional case reports of neurotoxicity on the combination, although generally well tolerated.
Succinylcholine	Effects have been prolonged.
Thiazides	Lithium clearance decreases. Lithium levels increase. As a rule of thumb: 500 mg of chlorothiazide will lead to a 40% increase in lithium level; 1 g a 70% increase.
Nonsteroidal anti-inflammatory agents	Reduce lithium clearance and increase lithium levels. Sulindac appears to be an exception.[b]

Sources. [a]Ghadirian AM, Annable L, Belanger MC: "Lithium, Benzodiazepines and Sexual Function in Bipolar Patients." *American Journal of Psychiatry* 149:801–805, 1992. [b]Ragheb M: "The Clinical Significance of Lithium-Nonsteroidal Anti-Inflammatory Drug Interactions." *Journal of Clinical Psychopharmacology* 10:350–354, 1990.

being used increasingly in psychiatry, primarily as an alternative to lithium. Beneficial behavioral effects were noted in seizure patients who received the drug, but it was not apparent if this was secondary to replacing more toxic anticonvulsants or a direct psychotropic effect. Controlled trials now indicate that carbamazepine has a therapeutic profile very like lithium's; it is an effective agent for treating mania and for the prophylaxis of recurrent unipolar and bipolar disorder. It also has some (lesser) value in the treatment of depression. Preliminary data indicate that it may have some role in the treatment of aggression.

Indications

Mania

When used in the usual anticonvulsant doses, carbamazepine demonstrates comparable efficacy to chlorpromazine and lithium (24, 25). As with lithium, there may be a delay of 7–10 days before the full impact is apparent. Combination with an antipsychotic leads to greater effect than either drug alone (26). The likelihood of response seems as great whether or not the patient has an abnormal electroencephalogram. There are suggestions that patients who cycle rapidly (more than three episodes annually) are more likely to respond to carbamazepine, but this may be an artifact of the patients who were studied initially. It is clear that some patients may respond to carbamazepine but not lithium and vice versa. The majority of patients will respond to both. Selection between the two is somewhat arbitrary. Lithium has frequent, generally mild side effects; carbamazepine rarely has toxicity, but it does carry the risk of one very unusual, very devastating problem—aplastic anemia.

Depression

In a study of 35 patients with depression, many of them with bipolar disease, one-third responded significantly and 20 had at least mild improvement while taking carbamazepine (27). These data are comparable with the impact of lithium.

Prophylactic Use

Published data largely report on lithium-refractory patients, a rather skewed, difficult population, but even with this group there seems to be a positive impact of carbamazepine (28, 29). Carbamazepine's effects are relative and not absolute; there is a decrease in the frequency, severity, and duration of episodes, but breakthroughs can occur. There are not yet good data correlating dose or level and response. The usual procedure is to aim for typical anticonvulsant blood levels of 8–12 µg/ml.

Violence

There is a growing literature, largely uncontrolled, studying the impact of carbamazepine on violence among patients with schizophrenia. All studies done so far looked at carbamazepine as an adjunct to antipsychotics. The preliminary results are sufficiently exciting to warrant adjunctive use of carbamazepine for this indication. This topic is addressed further in Chapter 8.

Toxicity

A skin rash is seen in 10%–15% of patients and is cause for discontinuation. Overly rapid escalations in dose are associated with decreased coordination, drowsiness, dizziness, slurred speech, and ataxia. These can be avoided by starting the drug slowly. Because it is a tricyclic, carbamazepine shares all the advantages and liabilities possessed by other HCAs in terms of cardiac impact.

A transient leukopenia, with up to a 25% decrease in the white blood cell count, occurs in 10% of patients. A smaller percentage may have this condition persist as long as they are on the drug. This is not an indication for discontinuation. There have been several case reports of isolated thrombocytopenia as well. In the first 18 years that carbamazepine was marketed, 20 patients developed aplastic anemia. Frequently fatal, this disorder causes suppression of erythrocyte, granulocyte, and thrombocyte formation. A hematologist should be consulted immediately if suspicions are raised of aplastic anemia. The estimated prevalence is less than 1 per 50,000 patients exposed (30).

Dosage

The usual practice for carbamazepine is to aim for anticonvulsant levels of 6–12 µg/ml. It should be started at 200 mg bid with an increase to three times per day after 3–5 days. The first level should be drawn 3–5 days later. Levels should be drawn 12 hours after the last dose. The usual effective dose is between 600 and 1,600 mg/day, divided into two or three doses. Signs of cerebellar dysfunction should lead to slower increases in dose.

Carbamazepine induces the enzymes responsible for its own metabolism. The effect of this is a predictable dip in level after 3–4 weeks of treatment. The physician should anticipate that an increase in dose will be necessary at that time so blood levels and clinical course should be closely monitored during this period.

Laboratory Monitoring

If the *Physician's Desk Reference* (PDR) recommendations were followed in full, the cost for a year's worth of laboratory tests for carbamazepine would have been $2,161 in 1982 (30). Much of the testing mandated by the PDR seems unnecessary. The primary fear is of aplastic anemia, but its onset is sudden and unpredictable and it is unlikely that frequent complete blood counts would prevent it; careful clinical assessment makes more sense. Patients should be instructed to monitor themselves for petechiae, signs of infection, and anemia (31).

Discovery of a white blood cell count below $3,000/mm^3$ or less than $1,500$ granulocytes/mm^3 should lead to discontinuation of carbamazepine. Table 4–5 contains suggestions for routine laboratory monitoring.

Hyponatremia can be associated with carbamazepine, so confusion or undue drowsiness are cause to monitor serum sodium levels.

Interactions

There are several case reports of neurotoxicity with patients coprescribed lithium and carbamazepine. These are balanced by many more case reports in which the combination was well tolerated. The added benefit of using both drugs has not been documented, although individual patients unresponsive to both agents

---

TABLE 4–5. **Carbamazepine laboratory monitoring**

- **Complete blood count with differential and platelets**
  At baseline
  At any sign of infection, anemia, or thrombocytopenia
- **Electrocardiogram**
  At baseline, if at risk
- **Serum sodium**
  With symptoms suggestive of hyponatremia
- **Carbamazepine levels**
  Every week for 4 weeks
  Every 3 months once stable

---

have responded to joint prescription (32). The more time-consuming, but prudent, course of action in a patient unresponsive to lithium is to discontinue it before beginning carbamazepine. If carbamazepine fails, either coprescription, valproate, ECT, or some of the alternative agents described in the next section should be considered.

The hepatic enzymes that metabolize carbamazepine are also utilized by a number of other medications. Some of the more important interactions are listed in Table 4–6.

■ VALPROATE

Another anticonvulsant, valproate, is emerging as an alternative for patients with bipolar disease. There is good evidence for its use in the acute phase of mania; however, it appears to be a poor antidepressant. There are no controlled trials of valproate as a prophylactic agent but in case reports it shows promise as a prophylactic agent for mania and perhaps for depression as well (33).

Preparations

There are four preparations of valproate on the American market. The best-studied and most commonly used form in psychiatry is an enterically coated compound, divalproex sodium (Depakote) that contains equal amounts of valproic acid and sodium valproate. This compound reaches peak levels in 3–5 hours, and its half-life is long enough to allow single daily nighttime dosing once steady state is reached.

Indications

Mania

If unselected groups of patients with bipolar disease are randomly assigned to groups given lithium or valproate, lithium emerges as the preferred agent (34). In contrast, when patients are selected based on intolerance or nonresponse to lithium, it is clear that a substantial number will respond (35). Some predictors are beginning to emerge about the type of patient who is more likely to respond to valproate (36). Patients with mixed states, dysphoric mania, rapid cycling, and electroencephalographic abnormalities are more likely to respond to valproate and less likely to benefit from lithium. It should be noted that these predictors are quite

TABLE 4 6 Important carbamazepine (CBZ) drug interactions	
● **CBZ decreases drug**	● **Drug increases CBZ**
Dexamethasone	Acetazolamide
(false-positive DST)	Cimetidine
Doxycycline	Danazol
Haloperidol	Diltiazem
Methadone	Erythromycin
Oral contraceptives	Propoxyphene
Theophylline	Valproate
● **CBZ increases drug**	(increases free CBZ)
False-negative pregnancy tests	Verapamil

Note. DST = dexamethasone suppression test.
Source. Modified from Ketter TA, Post RM, Worthington K: "Principles of Clinically Important Drug Interactions With Carbamazepine." *Journal of Clinical Psychiatry* 11:198–203, 306–313, 1991.

similar to the predictors of response to carbamazepine. Valproate is typically given in doses to achieve the low end of the usual anticonvulsant therapeutic levels or 50–125 µg/ml.

Depression
There is little reason to think that valproate is an effective antidepressant for any but the exceptional patient.

Prophylactic Use
There are no controlled trials, but there is a large collection of open trials that suggest that valproate may exert some preventive role. There is an indication that this role might be more impressive against mania than against depression (36).

Toxicity

Valproate is typically well tolerated; the most frequent side effects are gastrointestinal. The divalproex preparation is enteric coated and helps with this side effect. Most patients will accommodate to gastrointestinal difficulties. Hepatic toxicity occurs with some frequency in children, but is unusual in adults. Mild elevations of transaminase levels can occur. Hepatic fatalities have been confined to those under 10 years old with the exception of four adults on polytherapy (37). Approximately 10% of patients will experience some tremor. Other difficulties include alopecia and weight gain.

Dosage

Valproate treatment is usually begun with 500–1,000 mg/day in two to four divided doses. Acutely agitated patients may begin with 1,500 mg/day. Levels should be obtained 3 days after an increase in dose and the dosage should be titrated to between 50 and 125 µg/ml unless toxicity occurs. Once steady state is achieved the dose may be changed to a single nighttime dose.

Laboratory Monitoring

Liver function tests and a complete blood count with platelets should be obtained at baseline and repeated on a monthly basis for several months. Once stabilized, this testing can be limited to every 6 months, although there is a legitimate argument for relying on clinical monitoring alone (31).

■ CHOOSING AMONG LITHIUM, CARBAMAZEPINE, AND VALPROATE

Twenty to forty percent of patients with classical bipolar disease do not respond to lithium or are intolerant of it (38). Lithium remains the gold standard against which all other agents are measured. For patients with classical bipolar disease the choice is easy; lithium is the drug with which to begin. For patients who fail to respond to lithium, the choice is still easy. The data are stronger for selecting carbamazepine than for valproate; therefore, carbamazepine treatment is the logical next step, with valproate reserved for the patient who fails to do well with carbamazepine.

The more difficult problem is what to do with the atypical patient. Rapid-cycling patients, those with dysphoric mania, or patients with mixed-state bipolar disease are less likely to respond to lithium and more likely to respond to carbamazepine or valproate. An argument can be made for foregoing lithium with such patients.

■ ALTERNATIVE AGENTS IN BIPOLAR DISORDER

Clonazepam

Chouinard and co-workers performed a randomized, double-blind, crossover trial comparing clonazepam and lithium in acute mania (39). Daily doses ranged from 4 to 16 mg for clonazepam and 900 to 2,100 mg for lithium. The results were comparable. There are no data comparing the two drugs for maintenance treatment.

Calcium Channel Blockers

There are several small studies of verapamil and one of diltiazem. Verapamil has been used with daily doses ranging from 160 to 480 mg in patients with acute mania. There are no controlled trials of maintenance use. It has proved helpful in the limited numbers of patients who have been studied (40).

■ REFERENCES

1. Cade JFJ: Lithium salts in the treatment of psychotic excitement. Med J Aust 2:349–352, 1949
2. Gershon S, Goodnick PJ: Lithium use in affective disorders. Psychiatric Annals 11:143–153, 1981
3. Jefferson JW, Greist JH, Ackerman DL, et al: Lithium Encyclopedia for Clinical Practice, 2nd Edition. Washington, DC, American Psychiatric Press, 1987
4. Wehr TA, Goodwin FK: Rapid cycling in manic-depressives induced by tricyclic antidepressants. Arch Gen Psychiatry 36:555–559, 1979
5. Gelenberg AJ, Kane JM, Keller MB, et al: Comparison of standard and low serum levels of lithium for maintenance treatment of bipolar disorder. N Engl J Med 321:1489–1493, 1989
6. Faedda GL, Baldessarini RJ, Tohen M, et al: Episode sequence in bipolar disorder and response to lithium treatment. Am J Psychiatry 148:1237–1239, 1991
7. Consensus Development Panel: Mood disorders: pharmacologic prevention of recurrences. Am J Psychiatry 142:469–476, 1985
8. Delva NJ, Letemendia FJJ: Lithium treatment in schizophrenia and schizoaffective disorders. Br J Psychiatry 141:387–400, 1982
9. Zemlan FP, Hirschowitz J, Sautter FJ, et al: Impact of lithium

therapy on core psychotic symptoms of schizophrenia. Br J Psychiatry 144:64–69, 1984

10. Jefferson JW, Greist JH: Lithium carbonate and carbamazepine side effects, in Psychiatry Update: American Psychiatric Association Annual Review, Vol 6. Edited by Hales RE, Francis AJ. Washington, DC, American Psychiatric Press, 1987

11. Simard M, Gumbina B, Lee A, et al: Lithium carbonate intoxication: a case report and review of the literature. Arch Intern Med 149:36–46, 1989

12. DePaulo JR, Folstein MF, Correa EI: The course of delirium due to lithium intoxication. J Clin Psychiatry 43:447–449, 1982

13. Vestergaard P: Clinically important side effects of long term lithium treatment: a review. Acta Psychiatr Scand 67 (suppl):11–36, 1983

14. Franks RD, Dubovsky SL, Lifshitz M, et al: Long-term lithium carbonate therapy causes hyperparathyroidism. Arch Gen Psychiatry 39:1074–1077, 1982

15. Staner HC, Forbath N: Hyperparathyroidism, hypothyroidism, and impaired renal function after 10–20 years of lithium treatment. Arch Intern Med 149:1042–1045, 1989

16. Batlle DC, von Riotte AB, Gaviria M, et al: Amelioration of polyuria by amiloride in patients receiving long-term lithium therapy. N Engl J Med 312:408–414, 1985

17. Depaulo JR, Correa EI: Renal effects of lithium. International Drug Therapy Newsletter 20:13–15, 1985

18. Bendz H: Kidney function in lithium-treated patients: a literature survey. Acta Psychiatr Scand 68:303–324, 1982

19. Demers R, Heninger G: Pretibial edema and sodium retention during lithium carbonate treatment. JAMA 214:1845–1848, 1970

20. Guttmacher LB, Goldstein MG: Treatment of the cardiac impaired depressed patient, part two: lithium, carbamazepine and ECT. Psychiatr Med 6:34–51, 1988

21. Squire LR, Judd LL, Janowsky DS, et al: Effects of lithium carbonate on memory and other cognitive functions. Am J

Psychiatry 137:1042–1046, 1980

22. Faedda GL, Tondo L, Baldessarini RJ, et al: Outcome after rapid vs gradual discontinuation of lithium treatment in bipolar disorders. Arch Gen Psychiatry 50:448–455, 1993

23. Jefferson JW, Greist JH, Baudhuin M: Lithium: interaction with other drugs. J Clin Psychopharmacol 1:124–134, 1981

24. Okuma T, Inanaga K, Otsuki S, et al: Comparison of the antimanic efficacy of carbamazepine and chlorpromazine: a double-blind controlled study. Psychopharmacology 66:211–217, 1979

25. Placidi GF, Lenzi A, Lazzerini F, et al: The comparative efficacy and safety of carbamazepine versus lithium: a randomized, double-blind 3-year trial in 83 patients. J Clin Psychiatry 47:490–494, 1986

26. Klein E, Bental E, Lerer B, et al: Carbamazepine and haloperidol v. placebo and haloperidol in excited psychoses. Arch Gen Psychiatry 41:165–170, 1984

27. Post RM, Uhde TW, Roy-Byrne PP, et al: Antidepressant effects of carbamazepine. Am J Psychiatry 143:29–34, 1986

28. Fawcett J, Kravitz HM: The long-term management of bipolar disorders with lithium, carbamazepine, and antidepressants. J Clin Psychiatry 46:58–60, 1985

29. Post RM, Uhde TW, Ballenger JC, et al: Prophylactic effect of carbamazepine in manic-depressive illness. Am J Psychiatry 140:1602–1604, 1983

30. Hart RG, Easton JD: Carbamazepine and hematological monitoring. Ann Neurol 11:309–312, 1982

31. Pellock JM, Willmore LJ: A rational guide to routine blood monitoring in patients receiving antiepileptic drugs. Neurology 41:961–964, 1991

32. Kramlinger KG, Post RM: The addition of lithium to carbamazepine: antidepressant efficacy in treatment-resistant depression. Arch Gen Psychiatry 46:794–800, 1989

33. Calabrese JR, Markovitz PJ, Kimmel SE, et al: Spectrum of efficacy of valproate in 78 rapid-cycling bipolar patients. J Clin Psychopharmacol 12:53S–56S, 1992

34. Freeman TW, Clothier JL, Pazzaglia P, et al: A double-blind comparison of valproate and lithium in the treatment of acute mania. Am J Psychiatry 149:108–111, 1992

35. Pope HG, McElroy SL, Keck PE, et al: Valproate in the treatment of acute mania: a placebo controlled study. Arch Gen Psychiatry 48:62–68, 1991

36. McElroy SL, Keck PE, Pope HG, et al: Valproate in the treatment of bipolar disorder: literature review and clinical guidelines. J Clin Psychopharmacol 12:42S–52S, 1992

37. Dreifuss FE, Langer DH, Moline KA, et al: Valproic acid hepatic fatalities, II: US experience since 1984. Neurology 39:201–207, 1989

38. Prien RF, Potter WZ: NIMH workshop report on treatments of bipolar disorder. Psychopharmacol Bull 26:409–427, 1990

39. Chouinard G, Young SN, Annable L: Antimanic effects of clonazepam. Biol Psychiatry 18:451–466, 1983

40. Garza-Trevino ES, Overall JE, Hollander LE: Verapamil versus lithium in acute mania. Am J Psychiatry 149:121–122, 1992

ELECTROCONVULSIVE THERAPY

■ HISTORY

Other than malarial treatment for general paresis, there were no effective biological treatments in psychiatry before the advent of convulsive therapies. A false premise—that epilepsy and schizophrenia could not coexist—led Meduna to attempt to induce seizures. Originally pharmacological methods were used, but they were difficult to control. Finally, in 1938, Cerletti and Bini used electricity to trigger seizures. This turned out to be a far more predictable technique.

The dramatic efficacy of electroconvulsive therapy (ECT), the absence of alternative treatments, and the fact that psychiatry now had a reimbursable procedure all led to a period of overuse. ECT was primitively administered without any anesthesia, oxygenation, or modification of the seizure. Little was known about limiting the memory impairment associated with the treatment. The inability to modify the peripheral manifestations of the seizure meant that fractures were common. Since then there have been dramatic improvements in the manner in which ECT is administered and increased understanding of the conditions for which the treatment is and is not helpful. Unfortunately, these new perceptions have not been sufficiently shared with the public, whose only understanding of the treatment usually comes from such unfortunate portrayals as the movie *One Flew Over the Cuckoo's Nest*. The result is that most patients enter into treatment far more apprehensive than they need to be.

The pendulum has probably swung too far in the opposite direction from the early period of indiscriminate overuse of ECT. ECT is increasingly reserved for patients in private and university settings. Veterans Administration and state hospital patients receive it far less frequently. Usage of ECT dropped from its maximum in the 1940s and 1950s in part because of the advent of effective pharmacological interventions. The decline may now have leveled off. Simultaneously, there has been heightened academic interest. A journal, *Convulsive Therapy*, has appeared and the number of scientific citations to this topic has increased dramatically (1).

■ EFFICACY

Depression

Recently, the controlled trials comparing ECT with other agents in the treatment of depression were pooled (2). Table 5–1 summarizes their data.

The effects of ECT are clear. The surprisingly negative outcome for the patients taking monoamine oxidase inhibitors (MAOIs) reflects one large study in which low doses were used, but the remaining data are about as expected for hospitalized patients.

TABLE 5–1. **Controlled studies of electroconvulsive therapy (ECT) in depression**

	ECT		Comparison treatment		Estimated % advantage in efficacy for ECT
	R	NR	R	NR	
ECT versus simulated ECT	73	36	33	63	31
ECT versus placebo	138	22	69	86	41
ECT versus HCAs	169	26	152	75	20
ECT versus MAOIs	140	24	63	99	45

Note. R = responsive patients; NR = nonresponsive patients; HCAs = heterocyclic antidepressants; MAOIs = monoamine oxidase inhibitors.
Source. From Janicak PG, Davis JM, Gibbons RD, et al: "Efficacy of ECT: A Meta-Analysis." *American Journal of Psychiatry* 142:297–302, 1985.

It must be emphasized that these studies were only of acute treatment. ECT is the most efficacious therapy available for single episodes of depression, but does very little to prevent recurrence. Because depression is often a recurring disorder, patients should routinely have some sort of medication after their ECT series. The analogy would be to treat a depressive episode with an antidepressant, but to then abruptly discontinue the medication once the episode had improved.

Use of ECT as opposed to heterocyclic antidepressants (HCAs) for major depression is associated with shorter hospital stays (3). Three-year follow-up data indicate lower mortality for ECT than for antidepressant-treated patients (4). Six-month follow-up revealed fewer suicides and suicide attempts among patients treated with ECT than among patients treated with antidepressants (5).

Predictors of good response to ECT in treating depression are quite similar to those that augur well for antidepressants. Biological signs are correlated with a positive response to both. The presence of mood-congruent psychotic features is associated with a better response to ECT than to antidepressants or antipsychotics alone, although antidepressants and antipsychotics combined do almost as well (6).

Mania

ECT is effective in the treatment of mania, but its use has largely been supplanted by antipsychotics and lithium. It is now typically reserved for patients who fail to respond to medication (Table 5–2).

TABLE 5–2.   **Indications for electroconvulsive therapy in mania**

- A manic episode refractory to 3 weeks of antipsychotic alone or antipsychotic and lithium.
- An episode of mania with excitement so severe as to pose a risk to the patient.
- Bilateral electroconvulsive therapy should be used.

A randomized prospective trial comparing lithium and ECT in the acute phase of mania found the two treatments to be comparable (7). Both required several weeks for really significant impact. ECT patients who received lithium after their course of treatment were no more likely to relapse than were patients who received lithium throughout the trial. The most surprising result of this study was the ineffectiveness of unilateral, nondominant ECT. Originally, the trial included a unilateral arm, but this was dropped because of the ineffectiveness of the treatment (8). This is the only diagnosis to date in which unilateral technique has proved ineffective. Retrospective trials comparing ECT and antipsychotics in mania have found them to be comparable.

Schizophrenia

From 1938, when ECT was discovered, until 1955, when chlorpromazine became available, ECT was the sole effective treatment for schizophrenia. Since then the use of ECT for this disorder has declined dramatically. It is now reserved for patients intolerant of antipsychotics or as a last resort for patients who failed to respond to several antipsychotics or antipsychotics and lithium. A recent review noted that ECT alone was ineffective in chronic schizophrenia and that its efficacy was inversely proportional to the duration of the illness. When used, ECT should be combined with continued antipsychotics, because the combination is more effective than ECT alone. Unilateral and bilateral ECT have comparable effect (9). When ECT is used, far more treatment is required: the usual norms are 6–12 treatments for depression and mania, but 12–20 for schizophrenia. What impact ECT has on the long-range outcome is still a largely unresearched question. The clinical impression is that patients tend to relapse after ECT is given and that the procedure, at best, buys a year or two of clinical improvement.

The predictors of good outcome are listed in Table 5–3. The more a patient's symptoms resemble schizoaffective disorder, the better the outcome. The more positive symptoms the patient has,

TABLE 5–3. **Predictors of positive response to electroconvulsive therapy among patients with schizophrenia**

- Short duration of illness
- Episodic course
- Good functioning before illness
- Significant paranoid, catatonic, or affective features
- Positive symptoms

the better the outcome as well. However, some chronic patients lacking positive predictors do respond. They are rare and difficult to identify in advance, but a trial may be warranted, especially if it is understood that such treatment is a long shot.

Depressive Pseudodementia

Depressed patients often present with significant cognitive impairment as one of the primary features of their illness. Demented patients often become depressed. There can be, then, a continuum between depression and dementia. It is often impossible to ascertain where a given patient falls along this spectrum without making an assumption of depression and attempting to treat it. The alternatives for such a therapeutic/diagnostic trial are ECT and antidepressants. Either is justified, but ECT may be somewhat more rapid and is more definitive, given the greater efficacy (10). These patients should be treated with a unilateral, nondominant technique because this is least likely to exacerbate their cognitive difficulties.

Sleep deprivation represents a more rapid and benign diagnostic approach. Following a night of total sleep deprivation patients with primary degenerative dementia with depressive features will typically worsen, whereas those with depressive pseudodementias will usually improve, if only transitorily (11). Although this approach has not been well studied, this might represent a reasonable screening test before ECT in cases where there is diagnostic doubt.

Other Disorders

There are anecdotal reports supporting the use of ECT in a wide variety of other conditions, including obsessive-compulsive disorder, phobic disorders, substance abuse, chronic pain syndromes, and others. None of these uses are well supported scientifically.

■ PATTERN OF RESPONSE AND DURATION OF TREATMENT

Signs respond well before symptoms do; this means that others will notice the change before the patient does. Sleep and energy are valuable early indicators of response. Just as with antidepressant treatments, extra caution should be exercised during the period of recovery because the risk of suicide may actually increase before it gets better.

ECT treatments are typically given three times a week in the United States. The usual pattern is to see a brief antidepressant response after the second or third treatment, with gradually lengthening and more robust periods of remission as the series progresses. Figure 5–1 shows the prototypic pattern of response. There is, of course, considerable variation. Some patients may show nothing until the eighth treatment, then suddenly blossom. ECT should probably not be abandoned until a patient shows no response after 10–12 treatments.

One of the most difficult questions surrounding ECT is that of how many treatments to give. Some physicians arbitrarily treat on the basis of diagnosis, so that all depressed patients receive eight treatments. Others wait until improvement has maximized, then add two more. This has been studied and there is no merit to adding the two treatments (12). The most logical approach is to continue treatment until the patient has either plateaued or had a decrease in the rate of improvement. This presupposes that treatment is not being limited by toxicity.

Diagnosis does afford some crude guidelines. Most patients

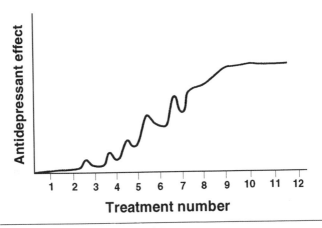

FIGURE 5–1.   **Response to ECT.**

with depression respond in 6–12 treatments, most patients with mania in a like number, and typical patients with schizophrenia in 12–20.

■ TOXICITY

There has never been much debate about the efficacy of ECT. The considerable controversy surrounding the treatment has largely centered around toxicity, especially the question of cognitive disturbance. Much of the debate has been based on emotion rather than science. The emotion should not be dismissed because it determines much of the climate surrounding the treatment. This had led to enactment of legislation in several states, such as California, so restricting ECT that it has sharply curtailed its use.

There is a very vocal minority of patients who feel ECT has severely damaged them. The majority of patients find ECT helpful and would repeat the experience. Only 18% of patients surveyed a year after ECT found it more upsetting than going to the dentist's office (13).

Mortality

The mortality associated with modern ECT is approximately 4/100,000 treatments. This is less than the risk of barbiturate-induced anesthesia alone (14). What deaths there are are probably cardiac in origin. Modern technique has substantially lowered the mortality. ECT should be performed in a setting in which cardiac monitoring is available and resuscitation is possible. If adequately trained personnel are present, the mortality would be even lower than the figure cited.

Brain Damage

ECT induces cerebral vasoconstriction. There is a transient increase in blood pressure and cerebral perfusion. Animals who are well ventilated do not experience cerebral anoxia. The older literature for both human and animal studies refers to punctate hemorrhages in brain, but it is likely that this represented agonal hypoxic change. There is a case report of an 89-year-old woman with bipolar illness who had 146 lifetime hospital admissions and in excess of 1,250 ECTs. After her death (unrelated to ECT), an autopsy was performed. Examination of the brain was entirely negative, except for changes consistent with aging (15). Imaging studies, including magnetic resonance imaging (MRI), have failed to show any change associated with ECT (16).

There is generalized electroencephalogram (EEG) slowing associated with ECT. This generally reverts to normal within 1 month of the completion of a series, but rarely may persist for 3 months or more. Slowing is proportional to the number of treatments. There is no clear correlation between either clinical improvement or memory impairment and slowing (17).

Depression itself is frequently associated with cognitive impairment. This often makes it difficult to separate the effects of the treatment from the impact of the underlying disorder. Many ECT patients experience an acute amnesic syndrome at the time of their treatment. There may be compromise in the ability to learn new information and difficulty in recalling data previously learned. These deficits are greatest for autobiographical information, especially for events that occurred around the time of the treatments.

The usual course is for the deficits to clear over the weeks after a series of treatments is concluded. Some patients report that they have persistent memory problems after ECT. Neuropsychological testing is not able to detect this, which may be more indicative of the insensitivity of the testing than of the absence of the effect. One potential problem is the reliance on mean or modal values; perhaps there is an impact, but this is only for a small subgroup of patients who become lost among the larger body of patients who are not impaired (18). Freeman and co-workers attempted to address this by advertising in a local newspaper soliciting patients who felt that ECT had irreversibly impaired their memory (19). Patients were more cognitively impaired than a control group. When use of medication and ongoing psychopathology were controlled, the patients who complained of memory loss were statistically more impaired on 2 of 19 tests used. If, instead, a prospective methodology is used focusing on the entire population of ECT patients, the deficits tend to disappear, although it may take patients 6 months to fully return to their baseline status (20).

For many patients, memory improves dramatically as depres sion resolves. One trial compared bilateral ECT with sham treatment in a depressed population. The simulated group had all aspects of the treatment except the passage of the electricity. Real, bilateral ECT acutely led to decreased concentration, short-term memory, and learning impairment, but improved remote memory. At 6 months no difference was apparent. Treatment-resistant patients, whether exposed to sham or real ECT, were significantly more likely to complain of memory impairment at 6 months (21).

Cognitive impairment associated with ECT has dramatically

lessened as technique has improved. Electrode placement is a major predictor of memory disturbance. There is substantially more impairment among patients treated with bitemporal stimuli than among those treated with unilateral positioning over the hemisphere nondominant for speech. Newer machines feature a brief-pulse waveform. Each stimulus consists of brief surges of electricity as opposed to the older sinusoidal current. The result is that far less electricity is required for seizure induction. The amount of current strongly correlates with confusion. Suprathreshold stimulation, or use of more than the minimal amount of electricity necessary to induce a seizure, will increase confusion. Patients with higher seizure thresholds, who are therefore exposed to more current, will experience more confusion.

Delirium is cumulative and proportional to the number of treatments in the series. Treatment more often than three times a week is associated with a denser delirium. Cognitive impairment can be minimized by using unilateral electrode placement, limiting the electrical stimulus, using a brief-pulse machine, treating no more than three times a week, and giving the minimal effective number of treatments. There is debate about whether some of these recommendations would impede efficacy. This is discussed in the section on technical issues.

Noncognitive Neurological Dysfunction

We recently reviewed the data from our institution and found that the mean blood pressure recorded within 1 minute of the seizure was 201/116; it reverts to normal readings within minutes. The hypertensive reaction is secondary to the outpouring of catecholamines that accompanies any seizure. Despite this response, cerebrovascular accidents are not encountered. Apparently very brief, but very impressive, hypertensive surges are well tolerated.

"Tardive" seizures, or spontaneous seizures occurring after ECT, are occasionally seen but they do not seem to occur more often than in the general population. ECT has even been used as a treatment for certain intractable patients with epilepsy.

Rarely, patients will have overly prolonged seizures with ECT. Seizures lasting longer than 5 minutes should be terminated with intravenous benzodiazepines or barbiturates. This is far more likely to occur with young patients or in patients who have an "irritable focus" (22).

Headaches are not uncommon for several hours after treatment. They typically respond to aspirin or acetaminophen. It is wise to give medication as soon as the gag reflex is intact for those patients who experience headaches on a repeated basis.

Cardiovascular Difficulties

We have recently completed a study of stable patients with high-risk cardiac histories, by virtue of past myocardial infarction, heart failure, or documented arrhythmia, who received ECT. All patients were taken off any medication that could affect cardiac rhythm. They all received 24-hour ambulatory electrocardiogram (ECG) monitoring for a day before and a day after treatment. Although we found significant rhythm disturbance, it was no greater after treatment than before (23).

A similarly high-risk population has been followed using serial creatinine kinase and serum glutamic oxaloacetic transaminase as markers of cardiac damage (24). No impact was seen. There is an increase in cardiac oxygen demand, associated with the increase in heart rate that is seen postictally (25). For this reason, it is probably wise to avoid ECT in the immediate period after myocardial infarction.

ECT may pose less risk than medication, particularly for those intolerant of antidepressants because of orthostasis, conduction disturbance, or arrhythmia. ECT has the advantage of placing the patient at risk only for a brief period, during which it is possible for them to be closely monitored (26).

If ECT is to be performed in a high-risk population, then extra precautions should be exercised. Patients should be cleared by a competent internist before treatment. Intravenous access should be maintained until the patient is fully recovered. The ECG should be monitored for 15 minutes before and after each treatment. There should be staff present trained in cardiopulmonary resuscitation, and the requisite equipment for the treatment of cardiac emergencies should be immediately available. Serum electrolytes should be monitored between treatments for patients on diuretics or digoxin, because hypokalemia can be associated with prolonged succinylcholine effect and digoxin toxicity. Hypertensive patients may benefit from pretreatment with a β-blocker or sublingual nifedipine (27). If a β-blocker is to be used, esmolol is preferred (28).

Miscellaneous Problems

Patients with *pseudocholinesterase deficiency* will have a very prolonged effect from succinylcholine. These patients should be ventilated until spontaneous respiration returns; at times intubation may be necessary. This disorder is genetic, so inquiry should be made about either personal or familial history of anesthetic misadventures. It is sufficiently rare not to justify routine testing.

   Myalgias occur in about 5% of patients. They are rarely very bothersome and are helped by aspirin or acetaminophen.

■ TECHNIQUE

The technique of ECT is well reviewed in an APA report issued in 1990 (29).

Informed Consent

For legal, ethical, and clinical reasons, it is vital that a full explanation of the treatment take place. Well-educated patients are less anxious about and more tolerant of treatment. Our patients are visited separately by the psychiatrist, the nurse who directs the treatment service, and the anesthesiologist. We have found tours of the treatment area for patients and their families to be helpful in allaying apprehension. There is a videotape featuring Max Fink, one of the real authorities on ECT, explaining the treatment for patients and their families (available from Somatics, Inc., Unit 16, 910 Sherwood Drive, Lake Bluff, IL 60044). All such efforts at education are to be applauded.

The ECT service at the University of Rochester Medical Center has developed a detailed consent form that incorporates, but modifies, the information recommended by the American Psychiatric Association Task Force on ECT (29) (Table 5–4). We were initially concerned that this amount of detail might be disquieting to patients, but have found the opposite to be the case.

The legal alternatives vary from state to state in terms of incompetent patients and ECT. One of the dilemmas is that patients with major depression are frequently imbued with profound hopelessness. They believe that no treatment can help them and extend this logic to include ECT. Other patients are convinced that ECT will kill them, although at the same time being able to quote the data on the risk of mortality. These patients, if suicidal, may readily consent because they look forward to death. Informed consent is, then, a thorny issue.

Physical Evaluation

With modified ECT, spinal X rays are unnecessary because spinal compression fractures are no longer seen. Routine laboratory studies should include an ECG; a chest X ray in those over age 35, in younger patients with a history of cardiac or pulmonary disease, or in smokers; a sequential multichannel autoanalysis-6 (SMA-6); and liver function tests. A thorough physical examination should be done. The only absolute contraindication to ECT is increased intracranial pressure, so focal neurological findings should prompt appropriate diagnostic studies to rule this out. Routine computerized tomographic scanning, MRIs, or EEGs in the absence of physical findings are not justified.

TABLE 5–4. **A consent form for patients being treated with electroconvulsive therapy (ECT)**

CONSENT FORM
Electroconvulsive Therapy

ECT has helped thousands of patients since 1938. It has been improved a great deal so that there are many fewer problems than there used to be.

Treatments are given in the morning before breakfast, about three times a week, by a psychiatrist, an anesthesiologist, and several nurses. While this is the usual schedule, your doctor may decide that some other schedule of treatments might be better for you.

You will be asked not to eat or drink anything after midnight on the night before treatments. In the treatment room you will be asked to lie down and you will be given oxygen through a face mask to help your breathing. Medicine which will make you feel sleepy will be given through a needle. You will also receive some other medicine, a muscle relaxant, through the same needle. As with any medicine, unexpected reactions might rarely occur. The treatment will be given while you are asleep. You should have no pain and will not remember the treatment. Two small round plates, called electrodes, will be held against your head and electricity passed through them. This will stimulate your brain and would ordinarily cause your body to shake and move strongly. The medicine you will have been given helps to protect you by almost completely getting rid of the shaking.

The treatment will take only a few minutes. You will awaken in the next room as if you were coming from a deep sleep. You may have some confusion as you are waking up. This usually goes away within a few hours. Nurses will stay with you until you are fully awake. Rarely, after the treatment some people may feel sick to their stomachs, have body aches, or headaches.

There are some other risks that could happen after the treatments. It may be hard to remember some things. You could have trouble remembering dates, the names of friends, or other facts. Normally this clears within four weeks after the last treatment. Very rarely aspiration leading to pneumonia can occur. Death is not very likely to happen. It has happened only once in every thirty thousand treatments.

The number of treatments you will have depends on how much they help you, but no more than 12 will be given without talking it over with you again. A second consent form would not be needed at that time if treatments were to continue.

(continued)

TABLE 5–4. **A consent form for patients being treated with electroconvulsive therapy** (continued)

You may stop the treatments at any time, but you will be asked to have as many as your doctor thinks you need. Feel free to ask your doctor or any of the ECT staff any questions that you may have.

I, _____, have read about the treatments, and they have been explained to me by _____ _____, who has also explained alternatives to ECT.

I agree to have treatments and anesthesia and understand that Dr. _____ will be in charge of my treatments.

Signature _____ Date _____

Before Treatment

Patients should have nothing to eat or drink after midnight to minimize any risk of aspiration. Treatments are given early in the morning in order not to prolong the fasting state.

At one time all patients received an anticholinergic before ECT. The aim was twofold: reduction of postictal bradyarrhythmia and of airway secretions. When carefully studied no difference was found between atropine and placebo in terms of secretions. Its use was supported for patients with hypotension or bradyarrhythmias before treatment, but not for others (30). If atropine is used, the usual dose is 0.4–1.2 mg im 45 minutes before treatment or a similar amount intravenously 3 minutes before the stimulus.

Patients should void before treatment to lessen the chance of embarrassing ictal incontinence.

The Treatment Team and the Treatment

ECT should be administered by a team consisting of a psychiatrist, an anesthesiologist, and a treatment room nurse. Another nurse will be necessary to monitor recovery if several patients are treated in succession.

The treatment room must contain an oxygen supply, a pulse oximeter, an ECG machine, a suction machine, a defibrillator, and other paraphernalia required for a medical emergency. An adjoining recovery room must be available if more than one patient is treated in any given session. Some programs choose to administer ECT in an operating suite where all of this equipment is readily available. Others find that such a setting is far more anxiety provoking for the patient. At our hospital we have chosen to make all this equipment available in the department of psychiatry and find that the familiar setting makes this inevitably frightening procedure much more tolerable.

The Anesthesiologist

The anesthesiologist should gain intravenous access and administer a short-acting barbiturate and succinylcholine. The barbiturate is given so the patient is asleep. If this were not the case, the patient might remember the onset of the inability to breathe induced by the succinylcholine, which is a terrifying experience. The barbiturate, typically methohexital or thiopental, is anticonvulsant, so the minimal effective dose should be used. This may be titrated by the absence of the blink reflex, elicited by stroking the eyelash. Once the patient is fully asleep, succinylcholine can be given. Succinylcholine leads to paralysis, preventing the peripheral manifestations of the seizure, but also suppressing respiration. The patient therefore must be ventilated. This can be done by either the anesthesiologist or the psychiatrist. Succinylcholine will cause fasciculations; once they are complete in the calf muscles, it is safe to proceed with the treatment. More reliable information is afforded by a nerve stimulator, a device that can be placed over the median nerve sending out a train of mild electrical charges that elicit movements in the hand. When these are no longer evident, the patient is ready for treatment.

The Nurse

The nurse in the treatment room should inflate a blood pressure cuff above systolic pressure on the right arm just before the injection of the succinylcholine and insert a rubber bite block before the stimulus. The cuff is intended to bar passage of significant amounts of succinylcholine into that arm. It is therefore possible to monitor largely unmodified seizure activity distal to the cuff. This poses no danger to the patient and, along with the EEG recording that should be obtained, offers confirmation that a seizure has taken place. If full modification occurs there may be no other evidence that this was the case. The cuff is placed on the right arm. Because the right side is controlled by the left cortex, right-sided motor activity after stimulation over the right hemisphere ensures that there was involvement of both motor cortices. Occasionally after unilateral stimulation, there is only contralateral activity. Such seizures are thought to be ineffective, and the patient should receive a second stimulus at a higher setting. The nurse's other, equally important, function is to offer support and reassurance to the patient.

The Psychiatrist

The psychiatrist is usually in charge of ventilating the patient and delivering the stimulus. Some teams choose to have the anesthesiologist manage ventilation instead. The patient is ventilated through the use of 100% oxygen delivered through a bag. The patient should be hyperventilated before the treatment because hypocarbia is associated with longer seizure duration, and this in turn correlates with better outcome. Ventilating can be resumed right after the stimulus, but the rate should be slower because respiratory drive will be triggered by the P_{CO_2} returning to normal.

The Treatment

The EEG should be monitored. If a unilateral stimulus is used, then following the same logic as the blood pressure cuff, the recording electrodes should be placed over the contralateral hemisphere (Figure 5–2). With bilateral technique they can be placed frontally. The seizure should be at least 25 seconds clinically or 35 seconds by EEG. Seizure duration by EEG measurement is always somewhat longer. Seizures shorter than 25 or 35 seconds are thought not to be antidepressant and restimulation should take place. The patient will be relatively refractory postictally so a higher setting should be used. Typical seizures are between 30 and 90 seconds.

Overly brief seizures are most probable with elderly patients. If this is the case, look to see if anticonvulsant medications are being used, notably benzodiazepines. If found, they should be discontinued. Stimuli that are right on the seizure threshold may lead to incomplete seizures, so the setting should be increased slightly. If all else fails, then caffeine sodium benzoate, 500 mg iv, may be given before treatment. This proconvulsant should both lower seizure threshold and prolong seizure duration (31).

The ECT machine should deliver a brief-pulse waveform because of the lesser amounts of electricity required. It should also have an impedance meter, which should be monitored to prevent skin burns from developing. There should be facilities for monitoring the EEG as confirmation that a seizure took place and that the duration was adequate.

Patients are typically asleep for 2–3 minutes, then awaken gradually. They should be turned on their side to prevent aspiration. Vital signs and consciousness should be monitored. They may return to their rooms when they are sufficiently awake as to be able to walk. They may find themselves somewhat sleepy for the remainder of the morning, but should be able to resume normal activities.

With improved technique, confusion has been minimized. This has allowed some patients to receive ECT on an outpatient basis. This is especially viable for patients who are receiving unilateral treatments and for those who have involved families who are able to drive them back and forth and stay with them for the duration of the treatment.

Electrode Placement and Settings

There is great debate in the field about the relative value of unilateral and bilateral stimuli. There is no quarrel about the associated cognitive impairment; acutely it is clearly less with unilateral, but this difference is not evident with long-term follow-up. The debate is whether unilateral works as well as or as rapidly as bilateral.

There have been over 30 trials comparing unilateral with bilateral ECT. Many have failed to detect a difference in efficacy, a similar number have shown a trend effect favoring bilateral stimuli, and a few have achieved statistical significance favoring bilateral stimuli. Much of the conflict reflects variability in diag-

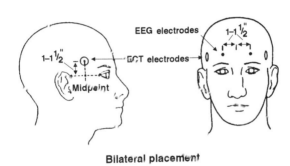

Bilateral placement

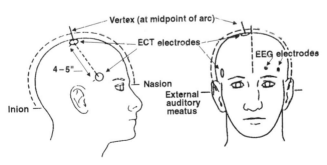

Unilateral nondominant placement

FIGURE 5–2. **Electrode placement.**

nostic and outcome criteria as well as problems in technique.

Unilateral ECT is somewhat more difficult to do well. The electrodes must be positioned more precisely and greater care must be taken to assure good contact between the electrodes and the scalp (32). The d'Elia position as shown in Figure 5–2 is preferred. With this approach one electrode is in a high centroparietal location, just to the right of the midline, and the other is placed over the right temple (33). If the electrode is not fastidiously positioned, there is the risk of establishing a current pathway that would bypass the motor cortex where much of the antidepressant impact might occur. The scalp must also be cleaned thoroughly with a saline solution just before treatment to ensure good contact.

There are also data implying that unilateral ECT is less effective if the dose is close to the seizure threshold (34). Very high dose unilateral ECT may approach bilateral ECT in efficacy, but then much of the cognitive advantage is lost (35). There is considerable variation in seizure threshold, although certain predictors are known. It is higher for elderly patients and increases across a series of treatments. Clinicians are faced with a dilemma: if unilateral stimulation is titrated down to the lowest setting that will induce a seizure, it is less effective. If pushed to a very high dose, unilateral stimulation will lose its advantage, which is lesser confusion, over bilateral stimulation. The usual compromise is to pick a moderate setting to begin with, but not to work assiduously at seeking the most minimal setting that will induce a seizure for unilateral treatments and to more aggressively seek the lowest possible setting for bilateral treatments. If the initial setting does not lead to seizure activity, then a second, higher stimulus should be given.

The conflicting data are hard to reconcile, but some attempt at compromise can be arrived at. Two leaders in the field, Richard Abrams and Max Fink, attempted to develop guidelines (36). They suggest that patients start with unilateral treatment unless there is an emergency, such as with acute suicidality or catatonia, or a past history of good response to bilateral ECT. Patients with mania should always be treated bilaterally. If, after five to seven treatments there are no signs of response, the patient should be switched to bilateral treatment. Any unilateral treatments should be given at a moderate, not minimal, setting.

■ ELECTROCONVULSIVE THERAPY AND MEDICATIONS

All patients receiving ECT should be off benzodiazepines because they raise the seizure threshold, resulting in shorter, less effective seizures, more treatments, and larger doses of electricity. This results in the patient's experiencing more confusion than is necessary (37). In addition, there are data indicating that concomitant use of benzodiazepines significantly compromises the efficacy of ECT (38).

MAOIs should be discontinued 2 weeks before ECT because they can lead to very prolonged apnea with succinylcholine (39). There is also concern that the catecholamines liberated by the seizure might lead to a hypertensive crisis.

Lithium also has the potential to prolong succinylcholine's effect and has been associated with more severe memory loss and atypical neurological findings (40). It should be discontinued 48 hours before ECT.

HCAs can be continued, but there is really no argument for doing so unless the patient will be going on the drug for maintenance. Even in such a case, it makes more sense to wait until the series is nearing an end before initiating treatment.

Antipsychotics combined with ECT in psychotically depressed or schizophrenic patients may lead to a more rapid response than ECT alone (41).

■ ELECTROCONVULSIVE THERAPY AND PHYSICAL ILLNESS

The only absolute contraindication to ECT is increased intracranial pressure. Space-occupying lesions in the brain, recent myocardial infarction, and some aneurysms are relative contraindications. Several conditions, including cardiac pacemakers and the need for anticoagulation, demand special cautions but can be managed safely. There are reports about the uneventful use of ECT in pregnancy (42).

Hypertensive patients may need to have their blood pressure brought under control before beginning treatment. Other patients who would be intolerant of the hypertensive surge postictally, such as patients who have had hypertensive cerebrovascular accidents, should be pretreated with β-blockers or sublingual nifedipine (27).

Epileptic patients can receive ECT, but their anticonvulsant medications may need to be adjusted. The most common problem is that the antiepileptic drugs raise the seizure threshold sufficiently to prevent seizures in these patients. In such cases their medication needs to be decreased enough so that they are responsive to treatment, but not so much that they have spontaneous seizures. Some patients with seizure disorder enter into status epilepticus with treatment. This problem should be treated as any other ECT-induced status. An appropriate intravenous benzodiazepine, such as lorazepam, should be kept available for such a situation.

■ MECHANISM OF ACTION

Chemical methods of seizure induction were effective but were much more difficult to manage in a reproducible fashion and therefore are no longer used. The obvious conclusion from this is that it is the seizure, not the electricity or the method of induction, that is important. Modification of the seizure with retention of the treatment's efficacy argues that it is something about the central impact that is responsible.

There is no correlation between memory impairment and antidepressant effect. Many patients have full recovery without any cognitive impairment. The obvious conclusion is that ECT works in some way other than causing patients to forget the source of their depression. Others have argued that ECT works by causing patients to feel as if they are being punished, thereby offering them a way to atone for their real or imagined sins. If this were the case, we would expect sham ECT to be far more effective than it is.

Just as with antidepressants, there is no satisfactory single explanation for all the data, but several arguments may eventually prove to be of value. There are animal data to support the thesis that ECT acts by inhibition of kindling. The kindling model makes note of the fact that repeated subconvulsive stimuli will eventually lead to spontaneous seizure activity. ECT, like carbamazepine, is a potent inhibitor of kindling in the amygdala and may act by virtue of being anticonvulsant (43).

Like HCAs and MAOIs, ECT downregulates the postsynaptic β-receptor. This does not happen acutely, but only after several weeks. This property is shared by all effective biological treatments of depression (44).

■ REFERENCES

1. Fink M: Is ECT usage decreasing? Convulsive Therapy 3:171–173, 1987
2. Janicak PG, David JM, Gibbons RD, et al: Efficacy of ECT: a meta-analysis. Am J Psychiatry 142:297–302, 1985
3. Markowitz J, Brown R, Sweeney J, et al: Reduced length and cost of hospital stay for major depression in patients treated with ECT. Am J Psychiatry 144:1025–1029, 1987
4. Avery D, Winokur G: Mortality in depressed patients treated with electroconvulsive therapy and antidepressants. Arch Gen Psychiatry 33:1029–1037, 1976
5. Avery D, Winokur G: Suicide, attempted suicide, and relapse rates in depression. Arch Gen Psychiatry 35:749–763, 1978
6. Parker G, Roy K, Hadzi-Pavlovic D, et al: Psychotic (delusional) depression: a meta-analysis of physical treatments. J Affect Disord 24:17–24, 1992
7. Small SG, Klapper MH, Kellams JJ, et al: Electroconvulsive treatment compared with lithium in the management of manic

states. Arch Gen Psychiatry 45:727–732, 1988

8. Small JG, Milstein V, Klapper MH, et al: Electroconvulsive therapy in the treatment of manic episodes. Ann N Y Acad Sci 462:37–49, 1986

9. Small JG: Efficacy of electroconvulsive therapy in schizophrenia, mania, and other disorders, I: schizophrenia. Convulsive Therapy 1:263–270, 1985

10. Allen RM: Pseudodementia and ECT. Biol Psychiatry 17:1435–1443, 1982

11. Buysse DJ, Reynolds CF, Kupfer DJ, et al: Electroencephalographic sleep in depressive pseudodementia. Arch Gen Psychiatry 45:568–575, 1988

12. Barton JL, Mehta S, Snaith RP: The prophylactic value of extra ECT in depressive illness. Acta Psychiatr Scand 49:386–392, 1972

13. Freeman CPL, Kendell RE: ECT, I: patients' experiences and attitudes. Br J Psychiatry 137:8–16, 1980

14. Fink M: Convulsive Therapy: Theory and Practice. New York, Raven, 1979

15. Lippmann S, Manshadi M, Wehry M, et al: 1,250 electroconvulsive treatments without evidence of brain injury. Br J Psychiatry 147:203–204, 1985

16. Coffey CE, Weiner RD, Djang WT, et al: Brain anatomic effects of electroconvulsive therapy: a prospective magnetic resonance imaging study. Arch Gen Psychiatry 48:1013–1021, 1991

17. Weiner RD: The persistence of electroconvulsive therapy–induced changes in the electroencephalogram. J Nerv Ment Dis 168:224–228, 1980

18. Weiner RD: Does electroconvulsive therapy cause brain damage? The Behavioral and Brain Sciences 7:1–53, 1984

19. Freeman CPL, Weeks D, Kendall RE: ECT, II: patients who complain. Br J Psychiatry 137:17–25, 1980

20. Taylor JR, Tompkins R, Demers R, et al: Electroconvulsive therapy and memory dysfunction: is there evidence for prolonged defects? Biol Psychiatry 17:1169–1193, 1982

21. Frith CD, Stevens M, Johnstone EC: Effects of ECT and depression on various aspects of memory. Br J Psychiatry 142:610–617, 1983

22. Guttmacher LB, Cretella H: The use of electroconvulsive therapy with three adolescents and one child. J Clin Psychiatry 49:20–23, 1988

23. Guttmacher LB, Greenland P: Effects of electroconvulsive therapy on the electrocardiogram in geriatric patients with stable cardiovascular diseases. Convulsive Therapy 6:5–12, 1990

24. Dec GW, Stern TA, Welch C: The effects of electroconvulsive therapy on serial electrocardiograms and serum cardiac enzyme values: a prospective study of depressed hospitalized inpatients. JAMA 253:2525–2529, 1985

25. Mulgaokar GD, Dauchot PJ, Duffy JP, et al: Noninvasive assessment of electroconvulsive-induced changes in cardiac function. J Clin Psychiatry 46:479–482, 1985

26. Guttmacher LB, Goldstein, MG: Treatment of the cardiac-impaired depressed patient, part II: lithium, carbamazepine, and electroconvulsive therapy. Psychiatr Med 6:34–51, 1988

27. Maneksha FR: Hypertension and tachycardia during electroconvulsive therapy: to treat or not to treat? Convulsive Therapy 7:28–35, 1991

28. Weinger MB, Partridge BL, Hauger R, et al: Prevention of the cardiovascular and neuroendocrine response to electroconvulsive therapy, I: effectiveness of pretreatment regimens on hemodynamics. Anesth Analg 73.556–562, 1991

29. American Psychiatric Association: The Practice of Electroconvulsive Therapy: Recommendations for Treatment, Training, and Privileges: A Task Force Report of the American Psychiatric Association. Washington, DC, American Psychiatric Association, 1990

30. Bouckoms AJ, Welch CA, Drop LJ, et al: Atropine in electroconvulsive therapy. Convulsive Therapy 5:48–55, 1989

31. Coffey CE, Figiel GS, Werner RD, et al: Caffeine augmentation of ECT. Am J Psychiatry 147:579–585, 1990

32. Weiner RD, Coffey CE: Minimizing therapeutic differences between bilateral and unilateral nondominant ECT. Convulsive Therapy 2:261–265, 1986

33. d'Elia G: Unilateral ECT. Acta Psychiatr Scand 215 (suppl):30–43, 1970

34. Abrams R, Swartz CM, Vedak C: Antidepressant effects of high-dose right unilateral electroconvulsive therapy. Arch Gen Psychiatry 48:746–748, 1991

35. Sackeim HA, Prudic J, Devanand DP, et al: Effects of stimulus intensity and electrode placement on the efficacy and cognitive effects of electroconvulsive therapy. New Engl J Med 328:839–846, 1993

36. Abrams R, Fink M: The present status of unilateral ECT: some recommendations. J Affect Disord 7:245–247, 1984

37. Stromgren LS, Dahl J, Fieldborg N, et al: Factors influencing seizure duration and number of seizures applied in unilateral electroconvulsive therapy. Acta Psychiatr Scand 62:158–165, 1980

38. Pettinati HM, Stephens SM, Willis KM, et al: Evidence for less improvement in depression in patients taking benzodiazepines during unilateral ECT. Am J Psychiatry 147:1029–1035, 1990

39. Marco LA, Randels PM: Succinylcholine drug interactions during electroconvulsive therapy. Biol Psychiatry 14:433–445, 1979

40. Small JG, Kellams JJ, Milstein V, et al: Complications with electroconvulsive treatment combined with lithium. Biol Psychiatry 15:103–112, 1980

41. Gujavarty K, Greenberg LB, Fink M: Electroconvulsive therapy and neuroleptic medication in therapy-resistant positive-symptom psychosis. Convulsive Therapy 3:185–195, 1987

42. Ferrill MJ, Kehoe WA, Jacisin JJ: ECT during pregnancy: physiologic and pharmacologic considerations. Convulsive Therapy 8:186–200, 1992

43. Post RM, Putnam F, Uhde TW, et al: Electroconvulsive therapy as an anticonvulsant: implications for its mechanism of action in affective illness. Ann N Y Acad Sci 462:376–388, 1986

44. Charney DS, Menkes DB, Heninger GB: Receptor sensitivity and the mechanism of action of antidepressant treatment. Arch Gen Psychiatry 38:1160–1180, 1981

AGENTS FOR THE TREATMENT OF GENERALIZED ANXIETY AND INSOMNIA

- **EPIDEMIOLOGY OF BENZODIAZEPINES**

Benzodiazepines (BZDs) are the most widely prescribed class of psychotropics. It has been estimated that 500 million people worldwide have had at least one BZD (1). During 1979, 11% of Americans between ages 18 and 79 received an anxiolytic; 1.6% of the population used these drugs every day during that year; 3.6% used them each day for a month or more. Long-term users were more likely to be female and elderly (2). Since 1979, American use has decreased by about one-third. The decrease probably reflects increasing awareness, by both physicians and the public, of the potential for dependence and abuse. Given that the first BZD, chlordiazepoxide, was not marketed until 1960, the amount of use is especially remarkable. Fortunately, the dramatic use of BZDs has been accompanied by a decrease in the prescription of barbiturates and meprobamate.

These drugs are prescribed much more often by primary care providers than by psychiatrists; only 10%–15% of the patients described above had seen a mental health provider in the preceding year. Either the primary caregivers are doing an excellent job of treating these patients, thereby obviating the need for a psychiatrist, or mental health providers are more reluctant to prescribe them, possibly because of their awareness of alternative forms of therapy. Many anxious patients will respond to relaxation techniques, insight-oriented therapy, or other nonpharmacological treatments. Given the potential toxicity of the BZDs, including dependence and cognitive difficulties, it is wise not to forget the therapeutic alternatives, especially if BZD use is to extend beyond a month or so. Unfortunately, there has been a tendency to line up in one of two camps with regard to BZDs. Klerman referred to this as representing a spectrum between "psychotropic hedonism and pharmacological Calvinism" (3). All too often it is based on the prescriber's value system rather than on science.

In 1989 New York State began to require that prescriptions for benzodiazepines be written on triplicate prescription forms in the same manner as narcotics. This was precipitated by the belief that BZDs represented a significant public health problem. Unfortunately, the chief result has been the substitution of other, more dangerous drugs (4). Similar moves are under way in other states. Although BZDs are at times abused, it is typically part of a pattern of polysubstance abuse. The usual patient takes less than is prescribed and for therapeutic, not recreational, purposes (5).

All BZDs are anxiolytics, sedatives, anticonvulsants, and muscle relaxants. The choice of which indication is to be submitted to the Food and Drug Administration for approval is partially a reflection of kinetics and partially of marketing strategy.

Knowledge of basic pharmacology has been of more use with the BZDs than other compounds. We understand the mechanism of action of the BZDs better than we do any other class of drugs. The kinetics predict the impact of these drugs very well.

This chapter addresses generalized anxiety disorder, but will not deal with obsessive-compulsive or panic disorders, which are discussed in Chapter 8.

■ BENZODIAZEPINE EFFICACY IN GENERALIZED ANXIETY DISORDER

Estimates of moderate or marked response based on controlled trials are about 35% for placebo, 50% for barbiturates, and 75% for BZDs. Efficacy is highest for those with severe anxiety. Those who are only mildly anxious will often feel that the sedation outweighs any benefit. The presence of prominent somatic features is associated with good outcome. Depression, interpersonal difficulties, and obsessive-compulsive features are all prognostic of a poor response. A previous good result with anxiolytics augurs well, as does a positive expectation of benefit on behalf of the physician. The outcome after 1 week of treatment strongly correlates with more long-term results. If no improvement is seen after the first week, the patient is unlikely to respond further. Maximal improvement is generally evident by 6 weeks of treatment (6).

There is little in the way of controlled data about the use of BZDs in acute, situational anxiety. What data there are indicate that acute anxiety is very responsive to a placebo. These patients have an expectation of improvement, and placebo or a BZD are therefore both associated with a good response. The difference between the two becomes apparent with more chronic anxiety.

■ DIFFERENTIAL DIAGNOSIS

The differential diagnosis for anxiety is quite long and requires the clinician to pursue a careful review of systems (7). Table 6–1 summarizes some of the main items to be considered.

Several items in Table 6–1 should be emphasized. A very careful history of substance use and misuse should be elicited, with emphasis on stimulants (including caffeine) and alcohol. A physical examination with special attention toward thyroid dysfunction and pheochromocytoma is clearly indicated. It should be remembered that akathisia can present as a poorly localized sense of anxiety with patients receiving antipsychotics.

The primary psychiatric differential diagnosis includes atypical depression, panic disorder, phobias, obsessive-compulsive disorder, and any ego-dystonic perception.

It is also important to remember that all anxiety is not pathological. Moderate amounts of anxiety often enhance performance. Treatment should be considered only when the anxiety bears little relationship to the stressor, when it is continuous, or when it restricts normal activities and functioning.

■ PHARMACOLOGY OF BENZODIAZEPINES

BZDs are rapidly absorbed from the gastrointestinal tract. Intramuscular absorption is quite variable and slower than after oral ingestion. The one exception is lorazepam, which has dependable and rapid absorption after intramuscular use (8). Midazolam, a

TABLE 6–1. **Physical causes of anxiety-like symptoms**

Type of cause	Specific cause
Cardiovascular	Angina pectoris, arrhythmias, congestive heart failure, hypertension, hypovolemia, myocardial infarction, syncope (of multiple causes), valvular disease, vascular collapse (shock)
Dietary	Caffeinism, monosodium glutamate (Chinese restaurant syndrome), vitamin-deficiency diseases
Drug-related	Akathisia (secondary to antipsychotic drugs), anticholinergic toxicity, digitalis toxicity, hallucinogens, hypotensive agents, stimulants (amphetamines, cocaine, and related drugs), withdrawal syndromes (alcohol or sedative-hypnotics)
Hematologic	Anemias
Immunologic	Anaphylaxis, systemic lupus erythematosus
Metabolic	Hyperadrenalism (Cushing's disease), hyperkalemia, hyperthermia, hyperthyroidism, hypocalcemia, hypoglycemia, hyponatremia, hypothyroidism, menopause, porphyria (acute intermittent)
Neurological	Encephalopathies (infectious, metabolic, and toxic), essential tremor, intracranial mass lesions, postconcussion syndrome, seizure disorders (especially of the temporal lobe), vertigo
Respiratory	Asthma, chronic obstructive pulmonary disease, pneumonia, pneumothorax, pulmonary edema, pulmonary embolism
Secreting tumors	Carcinoid, insulinoma, pheochromocytoma

Source.   Reprinted from Rosenbaum JF: "Anxiety," in *Outpatient Psychiatry: Diagnosis and Treatment.* Edited by Lazare A. Baltimore, MD, Williams & Wilkins, 1979. Used with permission. Copyright 1979, the Williams & Wilkins Co., Baltimore.

very short-acting agent used to induce anesthesia or for invasive procedures such as endoscopy, can be given either intramuscularly or intravenously, but is not available for oral use.

Metabolism

All BZDs except lorazepam, oxazepam, and temazepam are metabolized chiefly by hepatic oxidation. This process occurs quite slowly and leads to many pharmacologically active metabolites. Oxidation slows with age and hepatic insult such as that induced by cirrhosis. It is also vulnerable to other drugs that can inhibit the enzymes—notably cimetidine, disulfiram, and estrogens. The remaining BZDs are metabolized by glucuronide conjugation. The result is that the drugs that are conjugated—lorazepam, oxazepam, and temazepam—are less vulnerable to drug interaction, have no psychoactive metabolites, are shorter acting, and should be preferred in elderly patients.

Half-Lives

There is a marked difference in half-lives between single doses and steady-state kinetics. The drugs noted in Table 6–2 as having rapid onset are quite lipophilic. This facilitates rapid transit of the blood-brain barrier, but also results in a large volume of distribution. This in turn leads to a relatively brief duration of effect for a single dose because equilibration into the large fatty stores means that less drug is available acutely. This same process also means a very prolonged effect once steady state is reached because it takes a long time for the large volume of distribution to be cleared.

Take note of the half-lives listed in Table 6–2. Longer half-lives mean that accumulation is slow and extensive. It will take a long time to saturate the potential stores and to reach steady state. Washout of the drug will be similarly prolonged. Drugs with shorter half-lives will reach steady state much more rapidly but accumulation will be much less. Ninety percent of steady state will

TABLE 6–2. Pharmacokinetics of representative anxiolytics and hypnotics

Parent generic compound (trade name) and half-life	Clinically significant metabolites and half-lives	Approximate dose equivalence (mg)	Rapidity of onset	Cost to pharmacist ($)
Long acting				
Chlordiazepoxide[a] (Librium), 5–30 hours	Desmethylchlordiazepoxide, 5–30 hours Demoxepam Desmethyldiazepam, 36–200 hours	10	Intermediate	.03
Diazepam[a] (Valium), 20–100 hours	Desmethyldiazepam, 36–200 hours	5	Fastest	.02
Clorazepate[a,b] (Tranxene)	Desmethyldiazepam, 36–200 hours	7.5	Fast	.05
Flurazepam[a,b] (Dalmane)	Desalkylflurazepam, 40–250 hours	30	Fast	.07
Halazepam[b] (Paxipam)	Desmethyldiazepam, 36–200 hours	15		.31
Prazepam[b] (Centrax)	Desmethyldiazepam, 36–200 hours	7.5		.40
Quazepam (Doral), 25–50 hours	2-Oxoquazepam, 25–50 hours Desalkylflurazepam, 40–250 hours	15	Intermediate	.70

Intermediate				
Alprazolam (Xanax), 12–15 hours	4-OH-Alprazolam α-OH-Alprazolam Desmethylalprazolam	0.5	Fast	.52
Buspirone, 2–11 hours	5-OH-Buspirone	10		.91
Estazolam (Pro-Som), 10–24 hours	4-OH-Estazolam	2	Intermediate	.72
Lorazepam[a] (Ativan), 10–20 hours		1	Intermediate	.03
Oxazepam[a] (Serax), 4–15 hours		15	Slow	.25
Temazepam[a] (Restoril), 8–22 hours		15	Slow	.08
Ultrashort				
Triazolam (Halcion), 3–5 hours	α-OH-Triazolam	0.125	Fast	.49
Zolpidem (Ambien), 2 hours		10	Fast	1.75

[a] Available in generic form.

[b] Drug precursors that do not reach the systemic circulation in significant amounts without alteration.

Source. Modified from "Benzodiazepines: A Summary of Pharmacokinetic Properties." *Journal of Medicine* 306:401–440, 1982. Costs are average wholesale prices for the nearest available strength from *Red Book 1993: Annual Pharmacist's Reference* (Oradell, NJ, Medical Economics, 1993).

be reached by the time four to five half-lives have been completed (9).

The kinetics should determine which BZD is used for which purpose. An effective hypnotic should have a rapid onset of action; otherwise, the patient would have to either wait for several hours to feel the effect or plan well in advance on not being able to sleep. An as-needed (prn) anxiolytic should also have rapid onset. It should be noted that rapid onset is associated with a "rush" and increases the street value of an anxiolytic among drug abusers. Shorter durations of action are preferable in elderly patients for whom accumulation could be a problem. Also remember that all of the drugs listed are both anxiolytics and hypnotics, although they are marketed for only one indication. Lorazepam and alprazolam can be used as intermediate-duration hypnotics; flurazepam can be a long-acting anxiolytic.

■ INTERACTIONS

Cimetidine in particular, and disulfiram, estrogens, and alcohol to a lesser extent, have been known to inhibit the enzymes involved in oxidation, resulting in increased BZD levels for any given dose. The enzymes will be induced by cigarette smoking or heavy alcohol use, with lowered levels resulting. There is a report that coadministration of high doses of alprazolam and imipramine is associated with a significant increase in heterocyclic antidepressant (HCA) levels. HCA levels should be monitored if a BZD is also regularly taken.

The most significant interaction is that with alcohol and other central nervous system (CNS) depressants. The effects are additive. It is very rare to see a successful suicide involving BZDs that does not involve concomitant alcohol intake; coadministration turns a safe drug into a lethal combination. Patients should be cautioned about potential problems operating heavy machinery or driving if they are taking BZDs and not to have more than one drink.

■ TOXICITIES

Acute

Early in treatment, patients may be sedated, ataxic, or dizzy. These reactions are usually dose dependent and patients will accommodate to them with time.

Overdose

BZDs, unlike barbiturates, are remarkably safe drugs in terms of their potential as agents for suicide. Successful suicides almost always result from combination with other agents. The treatment of overdose is purely supportive, with the primary risk being from respiratory depression. Flumazenil, a competitive BZD antagonist, reached the market in 1992. Its chief role is to facilitate the diagnosis and rapid treatment of BZD overdoses.

Abuse and Dependence

BZDs are less valued by drug abusers than barbiturates. Abuse is most common as part of a pattern of polysubstance abuse, particularly among methadone maintenance patients who use them to augment methadone's effects and among cocaine abusers who attempt to alleviate the postcocaine "crash." Diazepam is generally preferred, probably because of its very rapid onset (10).

There has been long and heated debate about the potential for dependence associated with BZD use. Although patients almost never need escalations in their doses, there is little doubt that there is potential for psychological dependence and that physical withdrawal is seen. Serious withdrawal syndromes are seen after high doses for prolonged periods, but even conventional doses may have rebound anxiety after cessation. Withdrawal is generally better tolerated with the BZDs than with barbiturates. The half-life of the drug predicts much of the severity of the withdrawal syndrome. Drugs with very long half-lives tend to taper themselves. Drugs with very short half-lives generally do not reach steady state. The most dangerous withdrawals are seen with drugs whose half-lives are in the range of 8–20 hours, such as meprobamate, secobarbital, alprazolam, and lorazepam (11).

There is an identical withdrawal syndrome seen after prolonged use of high doses of alcohol, barbiturates, and BZDs. There is cross-tolerance between these agents, so that a BZD can, for example, be used to manage alcohol withdrawal. The syndrome is characterized at various stages by anxiety, insomnia, tremor, irritability, headache, hyperacusis, muscle twitching, hypertension, tachycardia, hyperreflexia, nausea, fever, depersonalization, hallucinations, major motor seizures, and even death. The severity of the withdrawal correlates with the duration and amount of exposure. Symptoms tend to be minor with less than 4 months of continuous treatment or with less than 30 mg of diazepam or equivalent daily. If patients have BZDs continuously for more than a month, then it is wise to taper the drug slowly. One approach is to decrease the first 50% relatively rapidly, to move more slowly for the next 25%, and then very slowly for the last 25%. Reports have indicated that residua of BZD withdrawal may be apparent as long as 6 months after discontinuation.

Rickels and Schweizer (6) have suggested that patients who are to be treated chronically with BZDs should have the smallest effective dose intermixed with periods off the drug. Such a program would prevent the development of physical dependence. Because the symptoms associated with the early phase of the withdrawal syndrome mimic those of anxiety, continuous use leads to a risk that patients will be maintained indefinitely on medication simply to counter the effects of discontinuing it.

Cognitive Effects

Short- and intermediate-acting BZDs have been associated with transient anterograde amnesia. Information is entered but not transferred from short-term to long-term memory stores. The cognitive impairment can be subtle but is sufficient that the physician should avoid short-acting benzodiazepines with cognitively compromised patients (12). Even cognitively intact patients exposed to typical doses of BZDs will show decrements in performance in tasks requiring attention, acquisition of new information, or such psychomotor skills as those required for simulated driving tests (13).

Behavioral Effects

Some patients, typically elderly and often with frontal lobe impairment, have BZDs prescribed for agitation and experience a paradoxical reaction with escalation of the targeted behaviors. This often leads to an increase in the BZD dose, further behavioral worsening, another escalation of dose, and so on. Remember that these drugs can make things worse as well as better (14). Depression is also a well-known, although rare, side effect of BZDs. It is more likely in patients with a history of affective disorder.

■ MECHANISM OF ACTION

The mechanism of action of the BZDs is better characterized than any other class of psychotropics. We know that there is a large receptor with specific recognition sites for the neurotransmitter γ-aminobutyric acid (GABA), for barbiturates and for BZDs. These act to open a channel for the chloride ion, which in turn alters the intracellular environment in the postsynaptic cell. The major importance of this is that very specific agonists and antagonists are being developed that may ultimately be of clinical use and also further our understanding of the mechanism of anxiety.

■ DOSAGE

Anxiety should initially be treated on an as-needed basis. Treatment should attempt to address the underlying cause of the anxiety through the use of various psychotherapeutic techniques. If behavioral and psychological interventions fail, it may, on rare occasions, prove necessary to move to the use of chronic BZDs. Such trait-anxiety patients should have therapy initiated with doses equivalent to diazepam 5 mg bid. Adjustments should not be made until steady state has been reached, usually at four to five times the half-life. It would be highly unusual for a patient to require more than the equivalent of 40 mg of diazepam daily and typically far less should be used. Table 6–2 lists dose equivalents for various BZDs. Similar doses can be used for acute, situational anxiety when brief treatment is necessary.

■ NONBENZODIAZEPINE ANXIOLYTICS

Antidepressants

In an interesting study, patients with generalized anxiety disorder who were not depressed were randomly assigned to either alprazolam or imipramine (15). Doses were varied depending on clinical response and ended up quite low (mean of 91 mg) for imipramine. Two weeks were required for imipramine to have any impact. By the end of the trial, both medications proved effective, with imipramine demonstrating a greater impact on the psychic manifestations and alprazolam a greater effect on the somatic symptoms of the anxiety. It should also be noted that many patients ended up preferring the alprazolam because of its ability to be used on an as-needed basis. More follow-up is clearly needed, but the implication is that HCAs might pose a nonaddicting alternative for patients with generalized anxiety.

Antihistamines

Antihistamines are really sedating, not anxiolytic, drugs, although hydroxyzine is occasionally prescribed for anxiety. There are no controlled trials to support such use.

Antipsychotics

Antipsychotics are reasonably effective anxiolytics, but their toxicity makes them an inappropriate choice for the treatment of anxiety given the other alternatives.

Barbiturates

There is no longer any role for the use of barbiturates in the treatment of anxiety. Overdoses are far more lethal, withdrawal is far more dangerous, and their potential for abuse is higher. The only indication for continued use is as an anticonvulsant, such as phenobarbital, or as an anesthetic agent, such as thiopental or methohexital.

β-Blockers

Many of the symptoms associated with generalized anxiety disorder are mediated by the autonomic nervous system. Some British psychiatrists have distinguished between "somatic" and "psychic" anxiety. Controlled trials indicate that diazepam is helpful with both the physical and cognitive aspects of anxiety. Propranolol is helpful with the somatic manifestations but does very little for the thoughts and feelings associated with the syndrome (16). There is one very interesting trial that found the combination to be more helpful than diazepam alone. Propranolol alone was less helpful than a placebo in this chronically anxious population. Propranolol's augmentation of the BZD was most apparent when there was adrenergic blockade as manifested by a reduction in the resting pulse rate by 7.5 beats or more per minute (17).

Buspirone

Buspirone (Buspar) is an azaspirone, structurally quite unique from other anxiolytics. Its primary advantage is its lack of toxicity.

Unlike the BZDs, it is relatively nonsedating, does not alter the seizure threshold, does not interact with alcohol, and is not a muscle relaxant. It does not interact with the BZD receptor and therefore cannot be used for withdrawal from CNS depressants. It seems to have little liability for abuse.

Buspirone is well absorbed after oral use, with much of the drug lost to first-pass effect. It is metabolized via hepatic oxidation. Its kinetics are not much affected by aging. The reported half-life has ranged from 2 to 11 hours in various studies. Patients with cirrhosis have a marked decrease in clearance, whereas renal failure has relatively little effect.

In chronic anxiety, buspirone's effect has equaled diazepam's when they are compared on a milligram-per-milligram basis. The onset of either is not apparent until after 1–2 weeks of treatment. Trials have not looked at truly acute, situational use. Unlike BZDs, buspirone is not effective on an as-needed basis. Typical dosing strategy is to begin with 5 mg tid, advancing by 5 mg every 3–4 days until maximal benefit is reached. Doses in excess of 40 mg daily have been associated with dysphoria (18). Four percent of patients reported an increase in nervousness that was significantly greater than with a placebo (19).

Although controlled-study data look promising, many clinicians are left with the sense that this drug has limited efficacy as an anxiolytic. Trials are now under way evaluating its role as an antidepressant.

■ TREATMENT OF INSOMNIA

One-third of Americans feel they have trouble sleeping; half of them consider the problem to be serious. One-tenth of that group, about 2% of the population, receive prescription hypnotics, and another 1% use over-the-counter hypnotics. A consensus development conference, sponsored by the National Institute of Mental Health, emphasized that insomnia is a symptom of heterogeneous origin and that every attempt should be made to address the underlying cause. Patients should be treated with the smallest effective dose for the shortest clinically necessary period (20).

The consensus conference also suggested that a careful sleep history be obtained, including detailed questioning about sleep habits, use of alcohol and medication, and underlying medical or psychiatric disorders. Obese patients who are heavy snorers may have the sleep apnea syndrome, which will worsen markedly with BZDs. Careful inquiry of sleep partners may be helpful here. They felt that hypnotics were most appropriate for those experiencing transient insomnia of several days' duration, such as during hospital admissions; for travelers; and for those with short-term insomnia lasting as long as several weeks resulting from situational stress. They noted that insomnia lasting longer than that was psychiatric in origin from one-third to one-half of the time, even if substance abusers were not included in the psychiatric population.

The consensus conference encouraged the use of nonpharmacological treatment. Table 6–3 lists some nonpharmacological approaches that may prove helpful. After these interventions have been exhausted, a short (less than 1 month) trial of hypnotics would be indicated.

The consensus conference suggested the use of a short-acting BZD as one alternative for transiently insomniac patients. Patients with short-term insomnia respond particularly well to the measures outlined in Table 6–3, but may also require hypnotics. If there is

---

TABLE 6–3. Nonpharmacological sleep aids

1. Decrease caffeine.
2. Eliminate alcohol and stimulant drugs.
3. Exercise several hours before bedtime.
4. Go to bed at the same time each night.
5. Avoid using the bedroom for activities other than sleep and sex.
6. Stay out of bed if awake.
7. Avoid daytime naps.
8. Consider relaxation techniques.

---

not significant daytime anxiety, then a short-acting BZD is most appropriate. Use should be intermittent with a night off of medication after a good night's sleep. If long-term insomniacs have a negative workup and no underlying cause can be determined, medication can be considered in combination with relaxation training and sleep hygiene techniques as outlined above. Their recommendation is for treatment approximately one night out of three, with the intervening nights available to assess progress. Intermittent use decreases the possibility of rebound insomnia, or a worsening of baseline insomnia seen after the discontinuation of hypnotics. This is more likely with long-term use and with long-half-life agents, but may exist even with one or two nights of a brief-duration BZD (21).

Choosing a Hypnotic

Once again, the kinetics should dictate the choice of a particular agent. Temazepam is marketed as a hypnotic but has a slow onset of action, generally making it an inappropriate choice. Triazolam has a very rapid onset but is of very short duration. It might be a better choice for a patient with initial insomnia than for another with midnight awakenings. Moreover, as noted above, there have been case reports of rebound anxiety on the day following very short-acting BZD hypnotics.

A number of other adverse behavioral reactions have been noted with very short-acting BZDs, including confusion, amnesia, bizarre behavior, agitation, and hallucinations. These are more likely at higher doses, with older patients, or when the drugs are combined with alcohol (22). As a result, therapy should be initiated with 0.125 mg if triazolam is to be used.

Lorazepam, not marketed as a hypnotic, would be a logical choice for an elderly patient, because of its rapid onset coupled with an absence of metabolites. Flurazepam would not be a good drug for elderly patients because of its very long half-life and potential for significant accumulation.

There is little reason to consider a non-BZD hypnotic, although many are available. Chloral hydrate is the alternative most often prescribed. The usual dose is 500–2,000 mg.

■ REFERENCES

1. Ayd FJ: Social issues: misuse and abuse. Psychosomatics 21 (suppl):21–25, 1980
2. Mellinger GD, Balter MB, Uhlenhuth EH: Prevalence and correlates of long-term regular use of anxiolytics. JAMA 251:375–379, 1984
3. Klerman GL: Psychotropic hedonism vs pharmacological Calvinism. Hastings Cent Rep 2:1–3, 1973
4. Weintraub M, Singh S, Byrne L, et al: Consequences of the 1989 New York State triplicate benzodiazepine prescription regulations. JAMA 266:2392–2397, 1991
5. American Psychiatric Association: Benzodiazepine Dependence, Toxicity, and Abuse: A Task Force Report of the American Psychiatric Association. Washington, DC, American Psychiatric Association, 1990
6. Rickels K, Schweizer EE: Current pharmacotherapy of anxiety and panic, in Psychopharmacology: The Third Generation of Progress. Edited by Meltzer HY. New York, Raven, 1987
7. Brown CS, Rakel RE, Wells BG, et al: A practical update on anxiety disorders and their pharmacologic treatment. Arch Intern Med 151:873–884, 1991
8. Greenblatt DJ, Shader RI, Franke K, et al: Pharmacokinetics and bioavailability of intravenous, intramuscular, and oral lorazepam in humans. Journal of Pharmacological Science 68:57–63, 1979
9. Greenblatt DJ, Shader RI, Abernethy DR: Current status of benzodiazepines. N Engl J Med 309:354–358, 410–416, 1983
10. Griffiths RR, Sannerud CA: Abuse of and dependence on benzodiazepines and other anxiolytic/sedative drugs, in Psychopharmacology: The Third Generation of Progress. Edited

by Meltzer HY. New York, Raven, 1987

11. Hollister LE: Clinical Pharmacology of Psychotherapeutic Drugs, 2nd Edition. New York, Churchill-Livingstone, 1983

12. Scharf MB, Saskin P, Fletcher K: Benzodiazepine-induced amnesia: clinical and laboratory findings. J Clin Psychiatry Monograph 5:14–17, 1987

13. Taylor JL, Tinklenberg JR: Cognitive impairment and benzodiazepines, in Psychopharmacology: The Third Generation of Progress. Edited by Meltzer HY. New York, Raven, 1987

14. Hall RCW, Zisook S: Paradoxical reactions to benzodiazepines. Br J Clin Pharmacol 11:91S–104S, 1981

15. Hoehn-Saric R, McLeod DR, Zimmerli WD: Differential effects of alprazolam and imipramine in generalized anxiety disorder: somatic versus psychic symptoms. J Clin Psychiatry 49:293–301, 1988

16. Noyes R: Beta-blocking drugs and anxiety. Psychosomatics 23:155–170, 1982

17. Hallstrom C, Treasden I, Edwards JG, et al: Diazepam, propranolol, and their combination in the management of chronic anxiety. Br J Psychiatry 139:417–421, 1981

18. Griffith JD, Jasinski DR, Casten GP, et al: Investigation of the abuse potential of buspirone in alcohol-dependent patients. Am J Med 80 (suppl 3B):30–35, 1986

19. Newton RE, Marunycz JD, Aldedice MT, et al: Review of the side effect profile of buspirone. Am J Med 80 (suppl 3B):17–21, 1986

20. National Institute of Mental Health Consensus Development Conference: Drugs and insomnia: the use of medications to promote sleep. JAMA 251:2410–2414, 1984

21. Kales A, Manfredi RL, Vgontzas AN, et al: Rebound insomnia after only brief and intermittent use of rapidly eliminated benzodiazepines. Clin Pharmacol Ther 49:468–476, 1991

22. Wysowski DK, Barash D: Adverse behavioral reactions attributed to triazolam in the Food and Drug Administration's Spontaneous Reporting System. Arch Intern Med 151:2003–2008, 1991

GERIATRIC PSYCHOPHARMACOLOGY

The elderly population is increasing rapidly. They pose a special challenge to psychiatrists for several reasons. The incidence of psychopathology increases in old age, but the presentation of psychiatric disorders may differ from that seen with younger patients. Older patients are often physically ill and exposed to a number of medications. The illnesses demand awareness of the impact of the physical difficulty on medications and vice versa. Differential diagnosis may become clouded by virtue of the somatic problems. This relationship between physical and mental illness often requires close collaboration between the internist or family physician and the psychiatrist. Age has predictable impact on kinetics by virtue of alterations in the organ systems involved in the various phases of drug disposition.

A number of generalizations about elderly individuals made in this chapter. Realize, of course, that there are some 80-year-olds with the mind and body of a person 30 years their junior. Those patients should be treated as if they were 50.

In taking the history of an elderly patient it is important to get all the usual data, but several points need to be expanded on. The family history is taken, in part, to obtain genetic data. It now should include several generations of progenitors and offspring. Elderly patients may have past psychiatric histories. A brief episode of hypomania 40 years before could have importance in assessing the risk posed by an antidepressant. Inquire carefully about drug exposure, including over-the-counter medications and alcohol as well as prescribed substances. The elderly are three times as likely to receive prescribed drugs as the general population. Over-the-counter use is increased sevenfold (1). Find out about long-established personality traits by talking to family members. These are often exaggerated with the onset of dementia and disinhibition.

■ PHARMACOKINETIC CHANGES WITH AGING

Table 7–1 summarizes the kinetic changes associated with aging (1–3). A review of some of the points made in Chapter 1 will further understanding of Table 7–1. Steady-state plasma levels increase with larger maintenance doses, absorption of higher percentages of the drug, longer half-lives, shorter dose intervals, and smaller

TABLE 7–1. **Pharmacokinetics and aging**

Phase	Change	Effect
Absorption	Gastric pH increases. Decreased surface villi. Decreased gastric motility and delayed gastric emptying. Intestinal perfusion decreases.	Little overall change. Absorption is slower, but just as complete.
Distribution	Total body water and lean body mass decrease. Increased total body fat, more marked in women. Albumin decreases, γ-globulin increases, α_1-glycoprotein unchanged.	Volume of distribution (V_d) increases for lipid-soluble drugs, decreases for water-soluble drugs. The free, or unbound, percentage of albumin-bound drugs increases.
Metabolism	Renal: renal blood flow and glomerular filtration rates decrease. Hepatic: decreased enzyme activity and perfusion.	Decreased metabolism leads to prolonged half-lives, if V_d remains the same.
Total body weight	Decreases.	Think on a mg-per-kg basis.
Receptor sensitivity	May increase.	Greater effect.

Sources. From Thompson TL, Moran MG, Nies AS: "Psychotropic Drug Use in the Elderly." *New England Journal of Medicine* 308:134–138, 1983; Greenblatt DJ, Divoll M, Abernethy DR, et al: "Physiologic Changes in Old Age: Relation to Altered Drug Disposition." *Journal of the American Geriatric Society* 30 (suppl):S6–S10, 1982; and Beattie BL, Sellers EM: "Psychoactive Drug Use in the Elderly: The Pharmacokinetics." *Psychosomatics* 20:474–479, 1979.

volumes of distribution. Clearance increases with a larger volume of distribution and a shorter half-life. Clearance and steady-state level are inversely correlated. This is logical because the more rapidly a drug is cleared, the less of it is available. Clearance is more meaningful than half-life. Lithium's half-life is prolonged in elderly patients, but this is partially compensated for by the decreased volume of distribution.

The volume of distribution increases for all psychotropics with the exception of alcohol and lithium. The decrease in plasma proteins can lead to a higher percentage of unbound, free drug. Free drug crosses the blood-brain barrier and is psychoactive. Remember, though, that present plasma levels assay total drug and may not accurately reflect the amount of the drug that is available. Plasma proteins are also affected by malnutrition, so they may be compromised in an elderly impoverished or malabsorbing patient.

A decreased clearance and a prolonged half-life mean that it will take longer to reach steady state and to stop the effects of a drug. Practically, this means that the clinician working with older patients must move more slowly. The intervals between dose changes must be longer. Similarly, it will take longer to see if a drug will have an impact. In addition, there are indications that a change occurs in the sensitivity of the receptor for many drugs. Benzodiazepines (BZDs) and lithium will have a greater impact at the same blood level in an elderly patient. Heterocyclic antidepressants (HCAs) may not. The net effect of all this is that the wise clinician begins with lower doses with elderly patients, takes longer before making adjustments, and persists longer before declaring the drug a success or a failure.

■ ANTIPSYCHOTICS

Antipsychotics may be used for all the same reasons that are valid in younger patients. In addition, they may be used for management of agitation in some patients with dementia.

These are lipophilic compounds that are tightly bound to

albumin and metabolized hepatically. The net effect is a large volume of distribution, a long half-life, and a low clearance. The evidence for increased dopamine receptor sensitivity is particularly compelling in patients with structural damage of the brain (4).

Even more than with young adults, toxicities must be taken into account when antipsychotics are chosen for older patients. Elderly patients are more prone to parkinsonian side effects, with the curious exception of dystonias, which are decidedly rare. The incidence of akathisia increases with age. This is dose related and more probable with high-potency drugs. If these reactions develop, the treatment is to lower the dose or to switch to a lower-potency agent. Anticholinergics should be avoided because elderly patients are especially prone to anticholinergic toxicity.

Be especially aware of the possibility of akathisia in a restrained patient. Patients with dementia tied into a gerichair because of agitation may be given an antipsychotic for the same indication. If akathisia results, the patient will become even more agitated because he or she will not be able to walk to discharge some of the anxiety. Increasing the dose of the antipsychotic will only increase the toxicity and worsen the situation.

The α-blocking property of some antipsychotics can lead to orthostasis, resulting in falls and broken hips. This risk increases with low-potency agents and with coprescription of HCAs.

Anticholinergic effects can exacerbate cognitive impairment and lead to delirium; constipation that causes impaction; urinary retention, especially in men with enlarged prostates; urinary tract infections; and visual blurring. These problems are most common with low-potency agents, especially thioridazine.

Phenothiazines, but not other conventional antipsychotics, have been associated with agranulocytosis, especially in elderly women. This is most probable in the first 2 months. Because of this, elderly patients exposed to phenothiazines should have baseline complete blood counts drawn. A close watch should be maintained for the possibility of infection. Phenothiazines may also be associated with a poikilothermic reaction in elderly patients.

The incidence of tardive dyskinesia increases with age, but there are a wide variety of senescent dyskinesias that can complicate differential diagnosis. A baseline Abnormal Involuntary Movement Scale (AIMS) examination should be performed (5) (see also Chapter 2, Table 2–6). Tardive dyskinesia is less likely to reverse among elderly patients.

Patients should start with doses that are 10%–25% of the usual younger-adult doses, beginning with something like haloperidol 0.5 mg qd to bid and then adjusting from there. Intramuscular doses should be avoided to whatever extent possible because the small muscle masses in older patients may make them quite painful. Lower-potency drugs are much more sedating, which may or may not be an advantage. The longer drug half-life in elderly patients will beget accumulation and considerable daytime carryover even if taken at bedtime. The choice of an agent should take this factor into account as well as the question of whether the patient is at greater risk from parkinsonian-like symptoms or orthostasis and anticholinergic toxicities. As with all other agents in elderly patients, doses should be adjusted less frequently than with younger adults.

■ ANTIDEPRESSANTS

Elderly patients have an increased incidence of depression compared with the general population. They are also more often prey to the many medical causes of depression, both idiopathic and iatrogenic. Because of this they should be very carefully reviewed for underlying physical disorder and medication status (6).

Heterocyclics

HCAs are bound to α_1-glycoproteins, which are less affected by aging than is albumin. The result is that the proportion of free drug should, in theory, be closer to that of younger people. These drugs are metabolized hepatically. Patients given amitriptyline or imipramine, which are tertiary amine HCAs, will demethylate them, yielding nortriptyline and desipramine, secondary amine HCAs. This process is slowed in the elderly, resulting in more of the parent compound. Table 3–4 in Chapter 3 shows that the tertiary amine HCAs carry more risk because they are more potent antagonists of the cholinergic and α-adrenergic receptors. Because we want to avoid these toxicities in elderly patients, it makes most sense to use the secondary metabolites. This choice is further supported by preliminary data for nortriptyline and desipramine indicating that the same blood levels associated with good outcome in younger patients probably operate in elderly patients. Thus, nortriptyline levels between 50 and 150 ng/ml and desipramine levels greater than 125 ng/ml seem to correlate with antidepressant response.

The variability in the efficiency with which hepatic metabolism occurs in these patients leads to poor interindividual correlation between dose and level. Generally much lower doses should be used, with initial doses of 10 mg of nortriptyline or 20 mg of desipramine being appropriate. If tolerated, the dose should be increased by the same amount after 5 days. A level can then be checked a week later unless there is clear indication of response.

Almost all of the potential toxicities discussed in Chapter 3 will occur with greater frequency in the elderly population. Orthostasis is the most frequent dose-limiting effect. Anticholinergic toxicity, as discussed with antipsychotics, is even more of a problem with HCAs. The delay with cardiac conduction can be a major problem. The lack of anticholinergic impact or effect on conduction often leads to the choice of trazodone, serotonin reuptake inhibitors, bupropion, or monoamine oxidase inhibitors (MAOIs). The serotonin reuptake inhibitors and bupropion do not cause orthostasis. Trazodone also is very sedating and can further ventricular ectopy.

Serotonin reuptake inhibitors and bupropion may offer some real advantage in terms of toxicity, and there are reasonable data on efficacy with elderly patients. Doses should be initiated at about one-half those given to younger patients (7).

Monoamine Oxidase Inhibitors

Because MAO activity increases with aging, there is basic science support for the utility of these drugs with older patients. Appropriate patients must be able to follow the diet or live in a setting that can guarantee adherence to the regimen. There are data supporting the efficacy of MAOIs in treatment-refractory geriatric patients. The absence of effect on cognition stands in contrast to HCAs and is particularly encouraging (8). Doses range from 15 to 75 mg for phenelzine and 10 to 40 mg for tranylcypromine.

■ LITHIUM

The indications for lithium are no different for older than for younger patients. Elderly patients are often on drugs, such as digoxin, thiazides, or nonsteroidal anti-inflammatory agents, that interact with lithium. They will typically respond to both lower doses and lower levels than younger patients. Levels that would be well tolerated by younger patients may lead to toxicity in the old.

Serum creatinine, a relatively reliable screen for renal impairment in the young, is not helpful in elderly patients. The loss of muscle that occurs with age means that a normal measurement of creatinine could occur at the same time there was serious renal damage. For this reason a 24 hour creatinine clearance test should be obtained before beginning lithium and every 6 months thereafter.

The possibility of sinus mode dysfunction is greater with elderly patients, especially if they are on a digitalis preparation or a β-blocker. Hypothyroidism is also more likely, as are parkinsonian symptoms. Lithium is a gastric irritant; an extended-release preparation may be better tolerated.

The decrease in the glomerular filtration rate and the volume of distribution with aging result in appreciably higher levels for any given dose. Patients in their 70s will require 36% less lithium to achieve a given level than will patients 50 years younger. This difference increases further with older patients (9). Moreover, elderly patients will respond to lower levels. Maintenance is usually accomplished with levels of 0.3–0.5 mmol/L, and acute treatment rarely requires levels greater than 0.8 mmol/L. Treatment is usually initiated with doses of 150 mg bid. Dose increments and reevaluation can occur every 5–7 days.

Several studies have reported on preliminary but promising trials of carbamazepine in geriatric patients. These studies included patients with hyperactivity and/or emotional lability associated with dementia (10, 11).

■ ELECTROCONVULSIVE THERAPY

Electroconvulsive therapy is often given to elderly patients. The indications and toxicities are discussed in Chapter 5.

■ ANXIOLYTICS

The major pharmacokinetic change with age relating to BZDs is an increase in the volume of distribution for all compounds and a slowing in oxidative metabolism. Conjugative mechanisms are relatively unimpaired so that the half-life for temazepam, oxazepam, and lorazepam changes very little, whereas the remaining BZDs are all significantly increased. This means that oxidatively cleared BZDs are much more likely to accumulate in elderly patients. When this is combined with increased sensitivity to the drug, as appears to be the case, the dangers become apparent. A study assessed risk factors for hip fractures, and as expected, HCAs and antipsychotics were implicated, presumably because of associated orthostasis and sedation. Long-acting, but not short-duration, BZDs were also found to increase the risk (12). This reflects the problem with accumulation.

Selection of a BZD should be based on rapidity of onset (which is a reflection of absorption and lipophilicity) and duration of effect. BZDs with short and intermediate half-lives are less likely to accumulate. Those drugs that are metabolized by conjugation are preferred because of their greater safety. Compounds with long half-lives, such as diazepam, chlordiazepoxide, or flurazepam, should not be used. The possibility of disinhibition with BZD use should be kept in mind. It is especially probable in cognitively compromised patients.

Oxazepam may be used in doses of 10–30 mg/day. It is usually initiated with 10 mg/day, with titration no more rapidly than every 3 days. Lorazepam is given in doses ranging from 0.25–1.5 mg/day, with the initial dose 0.25 mg/day. Both should be given bid or tid (13). These drugs may also be used as hypnotic agents, with some preference extended to lorazepam, which has more rapid onset.

Buspirone's kinetics are affected very little by aging (14). Limited data suggest that it might have some role with elderly anxious patients (15).

■ HYPNOTICS

Normal sleep architecture changes with aging. Phase advances are common, with elderly individuals retiring earlier and earlier. There are frequent midnight awakenings and compensatory daytime napping. Rapid eye movement (REM) sleep is distributed in shorter bursts and more evenly throughout the night. The very old and those suffering from Alzheimer's disease will have a reduction in the total amount of REM.

Sleep is further compromised by medical illness. Nocturnal angina may herald the onset of REM; chronic pain or paroxysmal nocturnal dyspnea may also awaken the patient. Institutionalized patients may be encouraged to go to sleep at a very early hour because of limited staffing on evening shifts. Daytime naps may lead to difficulties with nighttime sleep. Dementia is associated with significant worsening of sleep. Sleep apnea increases markedly from both peripheral obstructive and central sources. Nocturnal myoclonus will manifest itself as episodic twitches of the legs that occur intermittently through the night (16).

The first stage of treatment should always be non-pharmacological, with detail of a good sleep history. Daytime sleep habits, regularity of bedtime behavior, use of caffeine and alcohol, snoring, and nocturnal myoclonic jerks should all be inquired about. Good sleep hygiene habits should be encouraged (17) (see Chapter 6, Table 6–3). Hypnotics should be avoided in those patients in whom sleep apnea is suspected. In elderly patients, it is even more important to monitor daytime sequelae to hypnotic use. It should be remembered that no hypnotic should be prescribed on a nightly basis for an extended period. It is far more appropriate to use them 10–15 days out of the month, not allowing usage to extend beyond 1 or 2 months.

Unfortunately, there is a common belief that the antihistamine diphenhydramine (Benadryl) is a "mild" hypnotic. It is frequently prescribed for use on a nightly basis. It is also a potent anticholinergic, and patients are therefore exposed to anticholinergic toxicity. Nightly use also renders it ineffective for most patients within several weeks. Chloral hydrate is an old standard that is a more rational alternative to a BZD. It has a rapid onset, has a half-life of about 8 hours, and poses fewer problems in terms of interactions. The effective dose ranges from 125 to 500 mg. It is a gastric irritant.

BZDs remain the cornerstone of hypnotic therapy in elderly patients. Long-acting hypnotics should never be used because the possibility of daytime carryover is too great. Triazolam is cleared by oxidative metabolism but has such a short half-life that accumulation is not a major problem. Its chief problems are its delayed onset and the occurrence of amnesia in elderly patients. Because this appears dose related, therapy should be initiated with one-half of a 0.125-mg pill. Temazepam has a somewhat longer half-life but is cleared by conjugation. The absence of metabolites means that it is even less likely to accumulate with chronic dosing than triazolam. Because the program of intermittent dosing outlined above would prevent accumulation of either drug, they would both be viable choices. If, for some reason, they were to be regularly prescribed, temazepam would be preferred. Temazepam is best begun with 15 mg. Lorazepam 0.25 mg is yet another alternative.

■ TREATMENT OF AGITATION

Chapter 8 presents a more detailed discussion of differential diagnosis and the use of β-blockers and carbamazepine in the treatment of agitation. In mixed populations of patients with dementia, antipsychotics have a modest effect in terms of treating agitation and aggression. This, limited as it is, is greater than that of BZDs (18). There are no trials comparing antipsychotics with β-blockers or anticonvulsants. There is nothing to favor one antipsychotic over another, so prescription should be based on the criteria mentioned previously.

■ TREATMENT OF DEMENTIA

There is no treatment for the cognitive impairment of Alzheimer's disease. These patients may become agitated or depressed or have difficulty sleeping. Although we can address these behavioral concomitants, we cannot treat the primary disorder. Various nootropics, cerebral vasodilators, vitamins, and other nostrums have been advocated, but there is no real support for any such treatment. For now, we must await further research.

■ REFERENCES

1. Thompson TL, Moran MG, Nies AS: Psychotropic drug use in the elderly. N Engl J Med 308:134–138, 1983
2. Greenblatt DJ, Divoll M, Abernethy DR, et al: Physiologic changes in old age: relation to altered drug disposition. J Am Geriatr Soc 30 (suppl):S6–S10, 1982
3. Beattie BL, Sellers EM: Psychoactive drug use in the elderly: the pharmacokinetics. Psychosomatics 20:474–479, 1979
4. Salzman C: Clinical Geriatric Psychopharmacology, 2nd Edi-

tion. Baltimore, MD, Williams & Wilkins, 1992

5. Guy W: ECDEU Assessment Manual for Psychopharmacology (DHEW Publ No CADM 76-338). Rockville, MD, US Department of Health, Education and Welfare, 1976

6. National Institutes of Health Consensus Conference: Diagnosis and treatment of depression in late life. JAMA 268:1018–1241, 1992

7. Salzman C: Pharmacologic treatment of depression in the elderly. J Clin Psychiatry 54 (suppl):23–28, 1993

8. Georgatas A, Friedman E, McCarthy M, et al: Resistant geriatric depressions and therapeutic response to monoamine oxidase inhibitors. Biol Psychiatry 18:195–205, 1983

9. Jefferson JW, Greist JH, Ackerman DL, et al: Lithium Encyclopedia for Clinical Practice, 2nd Edition. Washington, DC, American Psychiatric Press, 1987

10. Leibovici A, Tariot P: Carbamazepine treatment of agitation associated with dementia. J Geriatr Psychiatry Neurol 1:110–112, 1988

11. Gleason RP, Schneider LS: Carbamazepine treatment of agitation in Alzheimer's outpatients refractory to neuroleptics. J Clin Psychiatry 51:115–118, 1990

12. Ray WA, Griffin MR, Schaffrer W, et al: Psychotropic drug use and the risk of hip fracture. N Engl J Med 316:363–369, 1987

13. Lawlor BA, Sunderland T: Use of benzodiazepines in the elderly, in Benzodiazepines in Clinical Practice: Risks and Benefits. Edited by Roy-Byrne RP, Cowley DS. Washington, DC, American Psychiatric Press, 1991, pp 213–227

14. Gammans RE, Mayol RF, Labudde JA: Metabolism and disposition of buspirone. Am J Med 80 (suppl 3B):41–51, 1986

15. Bohm C, Robinson DS, Gammans RE, et al: Buspirone therapy in anxious elderly patients: a controlled clinical trial. J Clin Psychopharm 10 (suppl 3):475–515, 1990

16. Crook TH, Kupfer DJ, Hoch CC, et al: Treatment of sleep disorders in the elderly, in Psychopharmacology: The Third Generation of Progress. Edited by Meltzer HY. New York, Raven, 1987

17. Consensus Development Panel: National Institutes of Health Consensus Development Conference statement: the treatment of sleep disorders of older people, March 26–28, 1990. Sleep 14:169–177, 1991
18. Salzman C: Agitation in the elderly, in Psychopharmacology: The Third Generation of Progress. Edited by Meltzer HY. New York, Raven, 1987

PSYCHOPHARMACOLOGIC TREATMENT OF SELECTED DISORDERS

■ AGGRESSION

Aggression may be a manifestation of disorders as diverse as paranoid schizophrenia, antisocial personality, and frontal lobe disinhibition. Whenever possible, the underlying cause should be treated, but there will be times when no clear etiology can be discerned or maximal treatment leaves violence untouched. For such patients, aggression may become a legitimate target in and of itself. This chapter discusses psychiatric patients troubled by chronic violence.

A body of literature is now beginning to evolve that focuses on violence as a target symptom. The patients who have been studied have varied widely. Studies have at times been flawed by heterogeneous patient populations. A wide variety of drugs have been used (1).

Antipsychotics

Antipsychotics are the drug of choice when violence results from a thought disorder. Aggression and hostility in schizophrenic patients are among the target symptoms that are most likely to respond. Unfortunately, all patients will not respond and other alternatives will need to be investigated. Patients who do not have thought disorders are unlikely to respond in any fashion except nonspecifically to the sedation. This does not justify the potential toxicity. Neuroleptics should not ordinarily be used for this indication with patients who are nonpsychotic. An exception can be made for some patients with dementia. This is discussed in detail in Chapter 7.

Benzodiazepines

There is little support for the use of anxiolytics in the treatment of chronic aggression. The primary benefit is sedation, which can be of considerable use when confronted with an acutely agitated patient, but there are few data to support chronic use. If used, a close watch should be maintained for behavioral disinhibition and worsening aggression.

β-Blockers

Most current research involves β-blockers. This is in response to a series of promising but uncontrolled trials involving patients usually defined by a wide variety of organic impairments including cerebrovascular accidents, developmental disability, and Huntington's disease, as well as schizophrenia. One controlled trial involved aggressive inpatients suffering from various organic brain syndromes. They responded significantly better to propranolol than to a placebo. The dose varied considerably, but the mean was 520 mg/day (2). Another study looked at violent psychiatric inpatients with multiple diagnoses. These investigators compared nadolol and placebo and found a statistically significant decrease in episodes of aggression without any change in the overall severity of illness (3).

Guidelines for this use of β-blockers have recently been published. Most studies have involved the use of propranolol, a lipophilic and therefore centrally active β-blocker. Asthmatic and diabetic patients and those with congestive heart failure or unstable angina should not be given β-blockers. Healthy patients can begin with 20 mg tid and increase the dose by a similar amount every 3 days. Once there is evidence of β-blockade as manifested by a pulse below 50 or systolic pressure below 90, then no further increases are indicated. This will typically be at doses of 800 mg or less daily. The dose should be maintained for 8 weeks or more to assess the impact of the medication. Concurrent α-blockers should be used with extreme caution because of the risk of hypotension. β-Blockers should be discontinued gradually because of the risk of rebound hypertension. Tapering should be no more rapid than 60 mg daily with the last 60 mg being discontinued in 20-mg increments (4).

In summary, the use of β-blockers in the treatment of aggression is promising but unproven. Patients with organic impairment are most likely to respond.

Carbamazepine and Other Anticonvulsants

Early and uncontrolled studies supported the use of phenytoin (Dilantin) in the treatment of episodic dyscontrol. Controlled, double-blind trials failed to replicate the earlier claims. This should serve as a caution in evaluating the more recent literature.

Carbamazepine has more support, primarily in the treatment of violent schizophrenic patients refractory to antipsychotics. The original report was from Finland where a group of extraordinarily violent and chronic schizophrenic women had carbamazepine added to their antipsychotics. The response was quite dramatic, with significant decreases in violence, amount of antipsychotic prescribed, and degree of restriction required (5). A later report approached being a controlled study. Luchins treated a group of similarly violent patients, all of whom had normal electroencephalograms (EEGs). When one patient developed fatal agranulocytosis, the study was discontinued, allowing a comparison of the 6 weeks before the anticonvulsant, the 6 weeks before discontinuation, and the 6 weeks afterward. Again, there was a significant effect favoring the drug. A second study by the same group showed similar results irrespective of EEG abnormality (6).

Lithium

Cade's original description of lithium's psychotropic effects suggested antiaggressive efficacy. Curiously, the best-studied population has been nonpsychiatrically defined prisoners. A double-blind, placebo-controlled study found that lithium maintained with levels in the 0.6–1.0 mEq/L range led to a significant decrease in major, aggressive infractions of prison discipline, but had only a minor effect on nonviolent transgressions (7). A similarly controlled study with aggressive developmentally disabled patients favored lithium over a placebo (8). There have also been many positive case reports with both organically impaired and psychiatrically defined patients. Lithium appears to have considerable promise as an antiaggressive agent but its target population, other than those with affective disorder, has yet to be defined.

In summary, lithium, carbamazepine, and β-blockers appear to be best for the treatment of aggression. The data are, at best, preliminary and the appropriate target populations have not been specified. It is not yet clear that aggression can be treated separately from the underlying disorder. The primary disorder should always be treated first, with these agents reserved either to augment the response or to treat patients who are refractory to more conventional therapies.

■ ALCOHOLISM

Disulfiram

Disulfiram (Antabuse) may be given to motivated alcoholic patients to decrease the likelihood of impulsive alcohol abuse. Within 12 hours of administration, disulfiram irreversibly inhibits aldehyde dehydrogenase, retarding the metabolism of alcohol and leading to increased levels of acetaldehyde if alcohol is consumed. Restoration of aldehyde dehydrogenase activity requires 6–7 days, so alcoholic patients need to plan a week in advance before drinking or risk a disulfiram-ethanol interaction. In its milder form, this reaction is characterized by flushing, tachycardia, tachypnea, a sensation of warmth, palpitations, and shortness of breath. If the alcohol exposure is higher, then it may progress to nausea, vomiting, a severe headache, and loss of consciousness. Fatalities have been reported because of myocardial infarction and cerebrovascular accidents.

Disulfiram's role is greatest in the first months of alcohol discontinuation. Older, socially stable, highly motivated patients are most likely to respond. It should always be part of a larger treatment program (9).

The usual dose of disulfiram is 250 mg/day. Its use has been associated with exacerbation of thought disorder and depression, a not unexpected effect, because it also inhibits dopamine β-hydroxylase, resulting in increased levels of dopamine and decreased levels of norepinephrine. It should not be prescribed for patients whose pulmonary or cardiovascular reserves are so limited that they have difficulty tolerating the alcohol-disulfiram interaction. The drug is metabolized via hepatic oxidation and should not be given to patients with advanced liver disease. The drug itself may be the cause of hepatotoxicity. It will interact with a number of drugs, decreasing the metabolism of oral anticoagulants, benzodiazepines (BZDs) that are metabolized oxidatively, and phenytoin. It may make patients drowsy and should therefore be given at bedtime.

Antidepressants

Among individuals who abuse alcohol there appears to be some benefit derived from antidepressant treatment during the first 3 weeks of withdrawal, if depressive symptoms, anxiety, and physical discomfort are the target symptoms. After that time there is no greater benefit than that afforded by a placebo. Interpretation of these data is complicated by the fact that almost all trials have suffered from low, possibly inadequate doses. Considerable skepticism is supported by the fact that because of hepatic enzyme induction, alcoholic patients require higher than normal doses of antidepressants to achieve therapeutic blood levels (10).

There may well be depression that is time limited during the first few weeks of alcohol withdrawal. A stronger case can be made for the use of antidepressants on an ongoing basis if the depression antedates the alcoholism.

Lithium

A somewhat more hopeful result was obtained in a well-designed study using lithium. Patients were randomly assigned to a placebo or lithium and followed for 1 year. They were also involved with Alcoholics Anonymous and an alcohol treatment program. Compliance itself, whether to lithium or a placebo, was helpful, but chances of abstinence were furthered by having a lithium level of 0.4 mEq/L or higher. Patients were as likely to respond whether or not they were depressed (11). Other well-designed studies have been less enthusiastic (12). The authors cautioned that the study was too preliminary to justify routine use of lithium in alcoholism treatment, but further study is certainly warranted. The data appear somewhat conflicting and will probably remain so until the relationship between alcoholism and affective disorder is better understood.

■ ALCOHOL WITHDRAWAL SYNDROME

Many different drugs have been advocated for the management of the alcohol withdrawal syndrome; all are based on the principle of finding something that is cross-tolerant with alcohol. The drug is then substituted for alcohol in sufficient amounts to avoid withdrawal and tapered to avoid the discomfort and dangers experienced with abrupt discontinuation. In recent years BZDs have been the cornerstone of therapy. They have the advantage of substituting readily for alcohol, offering sedation, affording minimal respiratory depression, and being anticonvulsant, thereby offering protection against "rum fits." This last quality makes BZDs preferred over antipsychotics.

Arguments can be made for various BZDs. Some clinicians

prefer long-acting drugs such as chlordiazepoxide, giving the patient a large-enough loading dose to suppress symptoms and then allowing the BZD to autotaper, thereby preventing later stages of withdrawal. Although this approach is elegant in its simplicity, there are problems. There is great potential for accumulation, especially in patients who are prone to hepatic insufficiency. The ideal drug is not affected by hepatic injury. Drugs cleared by conjugative metabolism are preferred over those cleared oxidatively because they are less affected by cirrhosis and there are not the problems of many metabolites and accumulation. Drugs that can be given orally, intravenously, or intramuscularly offer considerably greater flexibility. Lorazepam comes closest to satisfying these criteria and has an intermediate half-life (13). Titration of the dose to the patient's condition is vital no matter which agent is used. Alcohol withdrawal is sufficiently predictable that the dose can be adjusted on the basis of the patient's vital signs and other physical findings. Tachycardia, hypertension, and hyperreflexia should be prevented, and at the same time the patient should not be allowed to become overly sedated. Because of the wide variability between patients, it is impossible to offer any absolute guidelines about dose.

■ AMYTAL INTERVIEWS

Amytal Sodium, a barbiturate, can be given intravenously to disinhibit patients. It has been recommended as an aid to interviewing mute or stuporous patients, for distinguishing between organic and functional illness, and as a therapeutic measure to facilitate abreaction surrounding traumatic events, recovery of function in conversion disorder, and memory in patients suffering from amnesia (14). The results are often dramatic, and the efficacy of the procedure was unchallenged until a placebo-controlled trial was designed; a placebo emerged every bit as effective for all patients except those with catatonia (15). Another controlled trial, this time looking at patients with catatonia, found superiority for Amytal over placebo

(16). The positive response to placebo as well as to Amytal among noncatatonic patients presumably reflects the very high expectations for the procedure, which is customarily surrounded by a great deal of drama and expectations of "truth serum." In addition, it allows for a concentrated clinical interview and much attention to the patient. In essence, it underscores the value of a good placebo.

■ ATTENTION-DEFICIT DISORDER, RESIDUAL TYPE

A group at the University of Utah has developed diagnostic criteria and has been conducting a series of drug trials with this disorder (17). Required to make the diagnosis of this condition are the presence of attention-deficit disorder in childhood, persistent motor hyperactivity and attention deficits in adulthood, and two of the following list of symptoms: affective lability, inability to complete tasks, hot temper, impulsivity, and stress intolerance as an adult. Because of the medication response by children with this disorder, trials have proceeded with various stimulants as well as monoamine oxidase inhibitors (MAOIs) and bupropion. Methylphenidate was confirmed in a double-blind test as being quite helpful (18). Unfortunately, some subjects required frequent doses throughout the day because of the limited duration of action.

A recent open trial of bupropion was quite encouraging (19). Although a few patients were intolerant of even the lowest dose, the remainder all reported positive responses to the usual antidepressant doses. If confirmed in double-blind trials, these results would have considerable theoretical appeal because bupropion's longer half-life would obviate the need for frequent dosing and because of its lack of abuse potential.

■ COCAINE ABUSE

Preliminary data seem to indicate that antidepressants have a role in diminishing cocaine craving and depression after withdrawal.

Trials to date have focused on desipramine, chosen because, like cocaine, it is an adrenergic drug (20). Anecdotal reports also exhibit a role for imipramine. MAOIs have been advocated but probably should be avoided because relapse with cocaine, a potent pressor, when taking an MAOI could have dire consequences. Lithium, at least on an open, uncontrolled basis, has seemed helpful to those cocaine abusers with a history of bipolar disorder or cyclothymia. Pharmacotherapy should represent only one facet of a larger treatment program for cocaine abusers, just as for all other drug-dependent patients.

■ EATING DISORDERS

The distinction between anorexia nervosa and bulimia nervosa is underscored by the dramatic difference in response to pharmacotherapy. A study compared cyproheptadine (a serotonergic and histaminic antagonist), amitriptyline, and a placebo. In a 4-week trial, cyproheptadine, with a maximal dose of 32 mg/day, was both antidepressant and associated with weight gain in the restrictive anorexic group, but was associated with deterioration in the bulimic group. It was remarkably well tolerated in a population that normally encounters many side effects (21). This is the first drug that has been of benefit in a well-designed, controlled trial with this population.

In contrast, many agents have been helpful in patients with bulimia (22). Both heterocyclic antidepressants (HCAs) and MAOIs have assisted in decreasing the frequency of binges in patients with bulimia. This appears to be true irrespective of whether the patients were also depressed at the time of treatment. Trials with doses below the usual antidepressant range have been less effective. There are no trials directly comparing MAOIs and HCAs. Most studies have been short term; longer-term results have been conflicting. The results with intensive group psychotherapy would be expected to be more sustained than would the results of pharmacotherapy (23, 24).

■ OBSESSIVE-COMPULSIVE DISORDER

In almost all disorders it is safe to generalize that all members of an effective class of drugs are equally successful. Obsessive-compulsive disorder (OCD) is the exception to the rule. There is good support for clomipramine, fluoxetine, and fluvoxamine in the treatment of this disorder, yet other antidepressants have consistently failed. It appears that the common theme of success is inhibition of serotonin reuptake.

There are several unique issues in terms of pharmacologic treatment of OCD. Whereas placebo is helpful for some patients with almost all other psychiatric illnesses, it seems to have remarkably little impact on patients with OCD. Although treatment for OCD centers around the use of antidepressants, OCD exhibits several different features from depression. Patients with OCD who are not depressed are as likely as those with depression to respond. With patients with OCD and depression there is often a dissociation between the antidepressant and anti-OCD effects. The time course of response is often much more delayed than with depression. A good drug trial in OCD probably includes 10–12 weeks on medication.

Both obsessive and compulsive symptoms are responsive. The response is often imperfect with diminution in the frequency and intensity of intrusive thoughts and rituals. Behavioral treatment is especially helpful with compulsions and can reinforce the effect of the medication. Clomipramine is the best tested and is in many respects a typical sedating tricyclic (25). There is some increased liability for seizures; as a result there is a 250-mg/day maximum dose. Fluoxetine seems comparable in efficacy but needs to be administered in different doses than that used in the treatment of depression (26). The requisite dose is higher, with doses in the range of 60–80 mg/day required for antiobsessional effects. Fluvoxamine, another serotonin reuptake inhibitor not yet available on the United States market, has been similarly promising in controlled trials.

■ PAIN

Many chronic pain patients are significantly depressed. This can be both secondary to the pain and a cause of the somatic distress itself. Antidepressants have analgesic properties irrespective of the presence of depression. The onset of action occurs earlier and at lower doses than the usual antidepressant effect (27). Both serotonergic and adrenergic HCAs and possibly MAOIs have been shown to be of benefit (28, 29). Treatment has been effective both as the only medication and in augmentation of more traditional analgesics. A wide variety of chronic pain syndromes have been studied. Because there are few data supporting a relationship between dose and response and because many patients respond to very low doses, it appears prudent to begin with very small amounts (e.g., 25 mg/day) of imipramine or equivalent, with the dose titrated from there.

■ PANIC DISORDER

Patients with panic disorder often suffer from two kinds of anxiety: the panic attacks themselves and anticipation of the panic. The second type, which can be quite devastating, will frequently beget agoraphobia and other avoidant behaviors. Most HCAs, MAOIs, and several atypical BZDs are of benefit in treating the panic component. Once medication has prevented panic attacks, behavioral treatment is likely to be effective with the anticipatory aspect.

Controlled studies with HCAs have almost always used imipramine; all trials found it to be significantly better than placebo. A double-blind evaluation of trazodone found it to be without value, whereas imipramine- and alprazolam-treated patients did quite well in the same trial (30). There is little literature directly comparing various HCAs. One study found clomipramine preferable to imipramine (31). The controlled trials of MAOIs have been as positive as those with imipramine. There is support for the use of alprazolam from controlled studies, and several uncontrolled studies showing the positive effects of the BZD clonazepam. Trials of other BZDs have been either negative or equivocal.

Although MAOIs are effective, they are infrequently used as a first-line drug for this indication because there are other equally effective alternatives that do not require adherence to a special diet. That narrows the choice to an HCA, usually imipramine, or alprazolam or clonazepam. The BZDs have the advantage of having some minor effect on the anticipatory component and being somewhat less difficult to initiate. Imipramine is difficult to initiate but does not pose a problem in terms of withdrawal.

Patients with panic disorder are exquisitely aware of their bodies and are desperately searching for an explanation for their dysphoric somatic sensations. Some studies found the majority of patients unable to tolerate maximal doses of placebo because of side effects. HCAs cause some of the sensations usually connected with anxiety, including tachycardia, dry mouth, and light-headedness. Unless these problems are anticipated and discussed in advance, many patients have a difficult time tolerating the initial stages of imipramine treatment. Data are conflicting on dose and response, but it appears as if patients do best if full antidepressant doses are used (32). Because of the difficulty with compliance and initiating the medicine, I customarily start with a low dose of 25 mg and advance the dose more slowly than with patients suffering from depression. The same latency seen in treating depression occurs because most patients do not respond before 2 weeks.

Alprazolam or clonazepam are better tolerated in the beginning. Patients require substantially higher doses than they would for generalized anxiety disorder. Doses are usually in the range of 4–9 mg/day for alprazolam. The major liability is discontinuation. It is often difficult to distinguish between return of panic symptoms and BZD withdrawal. Panic disorder tends to be a chronic, unremittent disorder. Some patients do have spontaneous recoveries, nonetheless, so it is wise to slowly taper the drug every 6 months. Occasionally, patients can do without any medication. More often they are able to manage with a lower dose (33). Alprazolam is extremely difficult to discontinue because of its short to intermediate half-life. Clonazepam (Klonopin), another BZD, is normally used as an anticonvulsant. It has a longer half-life and poses less of a problem in terms of discontinuation. Studies have been entirely uncontrolled according to the literature, but some centers are using substantially lower doses, approximately 1.5–3 mg/day, with success.

■ PERSONALITY DISORDERS

Good clinical trials are rare primarily because of the diagnostic heterogeneity of patients subsumed under these labels. Recently some better studies have emerged. A series of trials from the National Institute of Mental Health indicate that carbamazepine is helpful with the behavioral dyscontrol and impulsivity sometimes seen with patients suffering from borderline personality disorder (34). Alprazolam, on the other hand, is associated with disinhibition and worsening of this problem (35). MAOIs may be somewhat helpful with the anger and hostility seen in patients with borderline personality. Antipsychotics seem to have limited utility (36). Carbamazepine seems helpful for patients with borderline impulsive disorders. In general it is safe to say that psychotropics have a relatively minor role and should be seen as adjunctive to psychotherapy (37).

■ PREGNANCY AND PSYCHOPHARMACOLOGY

Proving the null hypothesis, in this case that a drug does not cause problems for the fetus, is nearly impossible. There are a number of methodological problems, mostly relating to sample size. Malformations are rare events. To say that a drug does not double the chance of malformation may require a sample of 50,000. Moreover, an appropriate control group would be parents who are suffering from the same disorder but who are not receiving medication for it; otherwise, it is possible that the illness itself might increase the chance of malformation. Many mechanisms can be postulated, ranging from a common genetic locus to psychiatric disorder leading to inadequate antepartum diet and care. Things become even more complicated if we talk about anything other than congenital anomaly or miscarriage. Recently there has been interest in the idea of behavioral teratogens, or insults such as drug exposure during pregnancy manifesting itself later as behavioral disturbance in the child (38).

The only reliable system for implicating a drug is detecting an unusually high incidence of an otherwise rare anomaly and tracing it back to a common drug exposure in several mothers. This was the case with the hypnotic thalidomide, which led to phocomelia. The parents and their physician are often "caught between a teratologic rock and a clinical hard place" (39).

Unfortunately, those factors predictive of crossing the blood-brain barrier are the same ones that predict crossing the placenta. The time of greatest risk for the fetus is during the period of organogenesis from days 17 to 70 of the pregnancy. Some women are not aware of their pregnancy by day 17. Drugs that accumulate, as many psychotropics do, continue to exert their effect for a substantial period after discontinuation. This means that the possibility of pregnancy should be discussed in advance and good contraceptive practices should be encouraged. Use of psychotropics during the first trimester should be minimized to whatever extent possible.

Drugs taken later in pregnancy may affect the fetus through postpartum respiratory depression, neonatal jaundice, or hyperbilirubinemia. They might also induce fetal distress and premature deliveries. There is also the possibility of creating a withdrawal syndrome in the newborn.

Planned pregnancies are even more important for the woman

taking psychotropics than for other women. This is because of the risk that the medication might pose and the risk of pregnancy and the postpartum period on the psychiatric disorder. It is therefore vital that full discussion of contraception take place (40).

Pregnancy should not lead to automatic reflexive discontinuation of psychotropics. Instead there should be a reasoned assessment of the relative risk to mother and child of an untreated psychiatric disorder versus the risk the medication.

Antipsychotics

Dopamine blockade can induce menstrual irregularity. Patients need to be told that this is not a reliable form of contraception.

Offspring of individuals with schizophrenia have an increased incidence of congenital anomalies compared with the general population, but poor outcome appears to correlate more with severity of illness and chronicity than with medication exposure (41). No particular anomaly has been associated with the use of antipsychotics. Neuroleptic use late in pregnancy can lead to extrapyramidal syndromes and sedation in the neonate. Hyperbilirubinemia, neonatal jaundice, and hepatic enzyme induction have also been reported (42).

Lithium

Early data accumulated from an international registry of babies born after first-trimester exposure to lithium raised concern about Ebstein's anomaly, a rare cardiac malformation. This represents an example of recall bias; bad outcomes were disproportionately represented. Better data indicate that the risk of this malformation is quite low, well under 1% (43). Ebstein's anomaly can be detected by ultrasound and fetal echocardiography, and these tests should be routinely performed with mothers exposed to lithium during the first trimester of pregnancy.

If lithium is used, it must be remembered that there will be significant increases in both the volume of distribution and the glomerular filtration rate and that the dose will need to increase if the same level is to be maintained throughout pregnancy. Both will fall abruptly at the time of delivery, so it would be wise to decrease the dose just before the anticipated delivery. Lithium levels may be higher in the neonate than in the mother.

Anticonvulsants

Valproate and carbamazepine have emerged as reasonable alternatives for patients with bipolar disease. Evaluation of their risks in pregnancy is clouded by the fact that they are typically given to mothers with seizure disorders. It is difficult to separate the effect of the underlying disorder from that of the medication. It appears, however, that there is an increased risk of spina bifida. This is approximately 1.5% for valproate and 0.9% for carbamazepine (44). For this and other reasons, valproate and carbamazepine should not be used during pregnancy.

The first edition of this book suggested that carbamazepine might be a more logical alternative for pregnant patients with bipolar disease unable to function without a thymoleptic. Increased understanding of the rarity of Ebstein's anomaly and the risks associated with carbamazepine lead to a change in that suggestion; lithium has risks but is a viable alternative and is probably preferable to carbamazepine.

Electroconvulsive Therapy

The literature includes case reports of less than 100 patients who have received electroconvulsive therapy (ECT) in pregnancy. Most were in the second or third trimester and no problems were reported. The obstetrician should become a member of the treatment team, and fetal monitoring should be performed in advanced pregnancies. Although there are not a lot of data, it appears that ECT might be a reasonable alternative for some psychotic patients (45).

Antidepressants

There is a paucity of data on these drugs. An important recent study compared mothers with first-trimester exposure to fluoxetine, tricyclics, or nonteratogens (46). These investigators found a slight increase in miscarriage for both groups exposed to antidepressants and no increase in malformation. It is not clear whether the risk of miscarriage was associated with the antidepressants or with depression. MAOIs are prescribed sufficiently rarely that it is not possible to offer even tentative epidemiologically based conclusions. As a general rule, it is probably prudent to pick a medication that has been on the market for a while because there is probably more experience with it. Neonatal withdrawal from HCAs has been associated with dyspnea, difficulty in feeding, irritability, and urinary retention. Ideally, the drug should be withdrawn or the dose decreased before the patient's pregnancy comes to term.

Benzodiazepines

There has been debate about whether first-trimester use is associated with cleft palates. More recent data indicate that it probably is not. There are clear data on a BZD neonatal withdrawal syndrome. The maternal liver is better able to metabolize BZDs than is a neonate's, so it is probably preferable to taper the drug in utero rather than after birth (47). Animal studies with clinically relevant doses of diazepam in utero are associated with the development of behavioral difficulties, including chronic anxiety. There are few human data, but there is a suggestion of possible developmental delays (48). Because BZD use is usually less emergent than other psychotropics, it would be wise to avoid their use.

Breast-Feeding

Most psychotropics are excreted in breast milk. The amount varies, and we are typically unclear about how much of a given drug an infant can tolerate. Guidelines are generally based on supposition, although there are occasional reports of toxicity that can guide us more effectively.

Antipsychotics are passed into breast milk, but in low concentrations. There is no evidence of a clear effect on the infant. Lithium can appear in breast milk at one-half the concentration seen in maternal plasma. Lithium toxicity has been reported in breast-fed children, especially when dehydrated. It appears that both HCAs and MAOIs are excreted in such low amounts that they are safe for nursing mothers. Lethargy has been reported in nursing children exposed to BZDs; nursing mothers should avoid these drugs (49).

■ PREMENSTRUAL DYSPHORIC DISORDER

We are just starting to see the emergence of research literature about this disorder, which is termed "premenstrual dysphoric disorder" in DSM-IV (50) and was previously referred to as premenstrual syndrome (PMS). It is very important to distinguish this disorder from premenstrual exacerbation of other psychiatric disorders. This is not uncommon; for these patients the appropriate treatment is to treat the primary illness. If strict diagnostic criteria, including the need for prospective documentation over two menstrual cycles, are followed, the prevalence of this disorder falls below 5%.

Most studies of pharmacologic approaches did not include diagnostic criteria as rigorous as these and have ended up with very high placebo response rates. This has made it very difficult to establish that active treatment is more successful. Open trials with a variety of antidepressants have been promising. A recent trial with fluoxetine showed statistical significance over placebo (51). Unfortunately, this approach demands treatment throughout the cycle. Do not forget the very powerful impact of education in alleviating many of these symptoms.

■ SOCIAL PHOBIAS

Social phobias should probably be broken down into two forms: a discrete variant in which the patient has performance anxiety (often of public speaking, writing, eating, or drinking, or in men of urinating in a public rest room), and the more generalized variant in which any social interaction becomes quite anxiety provoking. This can be very disabling, with marked social avoidance and occupational impairment often resulting. Patients may experience panic episodes, but phobias are distinguished from panic disorder because patients with the latter condition will usually be somewhat reassured by the presence of others.

Performance anxiety is often quite responsive to β-blockers. Several placebo-controlled trials have looked at the impact of β-blockers on musicians or public speakers suffering from stage fright. A single dose (usually in the range of 10–40 mg of propranolol or equivalent) before the performance has enhanced both the quality of the performance and the patient's experience of it (52). Such use raised ethical issues because these are not absolutely benign medications. Patients who are asthmatic, diabetic, or prone to congestive heart failure should not use β-blockers.

More generalized social phobia can be quite disabling and is very responsive to treatment (53). There is good controlled-trial support for the use of MAOIs, typically phenelzine, in antidepressant doses (54). Open trials of buspirone, fluoxetine, and BZDs all show sufficient promise to warrant exploration with patients unresponsive to or intolerant of an MAOI.

■ TOBACCO DEPENDENCE

Cigarette smoking is a profoundly addictive behavior that is multiply determined. It is prompted by habit; thus it is often cued by daily activities. Unfortunately, cigarettes are often pleasurable and therefore reinforcing. In addition, tobacco is often used as a form of self-medication to counter withdrawal (55). Nicotine replacement systems effectively treat parts of the withdrawal system, successfully treating craving and dysphoric moods. They are less successful with hunger and weight gain. They should be part of a comprehensive smoking cessation program. The National Cancer Institute has materials available for both clinicians and patients (1–800–4CANCER). Six-month abstinence figures for patients treated with transdermal nicotine systems range from 22% to 42%, with the higher figures including a broadly based smoking cessation program.

There are two forms of nicotine replacement available. One is a gum (Nicorette) that allows patients to titrate their own levels by the number of pieces chewed and the vigor of their chewing. Some patients complain of the taste of the gum and others find it to be a gastric irritant; however, it does allow the patient greater control of the process. The other alternative is transdermal nicotine; several products are on the market. The data seem to indicate that the benefit of the patches occurs during the first 6–8 weeks. The strategy is to begin with the strongest patch available (typically 21 mg) and to continue with a new patch of similar strength each day for the first month, decreasing to the middle intensity for the next several weeks, and finally moving to the lowest strength (usually 7 mg) for the last weeks of treatment. Patients should be encouraged not to smoke at all at the beginning of this treatment.

Physicians should be cognizant of the high relapse rate and be prepared to continue working with the patient. Definition of which environmental cues, such as coffee drinking or driving, are associated with relapse is important, and appropriate substitutes should be found. The patches may cost several hundred dollars in pharmacy charges alone, but patients should be reminded about the cost of cigarettes. This is difficult, but potentially very rewarding, work.

■ REFERENCES

1. Tardiff K: The current state of psychiatry in the treatment of violent patients. Arch Gen Psychiatry 49:493–499, 1992

2. Greendyke RM, Kanter DR, Schuster DB, et al: Propranolol treatment of assaultive patients with organic brain disease. J Nerv Ment Dis 174:290–294, 1986

3. Ratey JJ, Sorgi P, O'Driscoll GA, et al: Nadolol to treat aggression and psychiatric symptomatology in chronic psychiatric inpatients: a double-blind, placebo-controlled study. J Clin Psychiatry 53:41–46, 1992

4. Yudofsky SC, Silver JM, Schneider SE: Pharmacologic treatment of aggression. Psychiatric Annals 17:397–402, 1987

5. Hakoloa HP, Laulumaa VA: Carbamazepine in treatment of violent schizophrenics. Lancet 1:1358, 1982

6. Luchins DJ: Carbamazepine in violent non-epileptic schizophrenics. Psychopharmacol Bull 20:569–571, 1984

7. Sheard MH, Marini JL, Bridges CJ, et al: The effects of lithium in impulsive aggressive behavior in man. Am J Psychiatry 33:1409–1413, 1976

8. Worrall EP, Moody JP, Naylor GT: Lithium in non-manic depressives: antiaggressive effects and red blood cell lithium values. Br J Psychiatry 126:464–468, 1975

9. Wright C, Moore RD: Disulfiram treatment of alcoholism. Am J Med 88:647–655, 1990

10. Ciraulo DA, Jaffe JH: Tricyclic antidepressants in the treatment of depression associated with alcoholism. J Clin Psychopharmacol 1:146–150, 1981

11. Fawcett J, Clark DC, Aagesen CA, et al: A double-blind, placebo-controlled trial of lithium carbonate therapy for alcoholism. Arch Gen Psychiatry 44:248–256, 1987

12. Dorus W, Ostrow DG, Anton R, et al: Lithium treatment of depressed and nondepressed alcoholics. JAMA 262:1646–1652, 1989

13. Rosenbloom AF: Optimizing drug treatment of alcohol withdrawal. Am J Med 81:901–904, 1986

14. Perry JC, Jacobs D: Overview: clinical applications of the Amytal interview in psychiatric emergency settings. Am J Psychiatry 139:552–559, 1982

15. Dysken MW, Kooser JA, Haraszti JS: Clinical usefulness of

sodium amobarbital interviewing. Arch Gen Psychiatry 36:789–794, 1979

16. McCall WV, Shelp FE, McDonald WM: Controlled investigation of the amobarbital interview for catatonic mutism. Am J Psychiatry 149:202–206, 1992

17. Wender PH, Wood DR, Reimherr FW: Pharmacological treatment of attention deficit disorder, residual type (ADD, RT, "minimal brain dysfunction," "hyperactivity") in adults. Psychopharmacol Bull 21:222–227, 1985

18. Wender PH, Reimherr FW, Wood D, et al: A controlled study of methylphenidate in the treatment of attention deficit disorder, residual type, in adults. Am J Psychiatry 142:547–552, 1985

19. Wender PH, Reimherr FW: Bupropion treatment of attention-deficit hyperactivity disorder in adults. Am J Psychiatry 147:1018–1020, 1990

20. Gawin FH: New uses of antidepressants in cocaine abuse. Psychosomatics 27 (suppl 11):24–29, 1986

21. Halmi KA, Eckert E, LaDu TJ: Anorexia nervosa: treatment efficacy of cyproheptadine and amitriptyline. Arch Gen Psychiatry 43:177–181, 1986

22. Walsh BT: Treatment of bulimia nervosa with antidepressant medications. J Clin Psychopharmacol 11:231–232, 1991

23. Mitchell TE, Pyle RL, Eckert ED, et al: A comparison study of antidepressants and structured intensive group psychotherapy in the treatment of bulimia nervosa. Arch Gen Psychiatry 47:149–157, 1990

24. Fairburn CG, Jones R, Peveler RC, et al: Psychotherapy and bulimia nervosa: longer-term effects of interpersonal psychotherapy, behavior therapy and cognitive behavior therapy. Arch Gen Psychiatry 50:419–428, 1993

25. Clomipramine Collaborative Study Group: Clomipramine in the treatment of patients with obsessive-compulsive disorder. Arch Gen Psychiatry 48:730–738, 1991

26. Pigott RA, Pato MT, Bernstein SE, et al: Controlled comparisons of clomipramine and fluoxetine in the treatment of obses-

sive-compulsive disorder: behavioral and biological results. Arch Gen Psychiatry 47:926–932, 1990

27. Magni G: The use of antidepressants in the treatment of chronic pain: a review of the current evidence. Drugs 42:730–748, 1991

28. Ward N, Bokan JA, Phillips M, et al: Antidepressants in concomitant chronic back pain and depression: doxepin and desipramine compared. J Clin Psychiatry 45 (sec 2):54–57, 1984

29. Davidson J, Raft T: Monoamine oxidase inhibitors in patients with chronic pain. Arch Gen Psychiatry 42:635–636, 1985

30. Charney DS, Woods SW, Goodman WK, et al: Drug treatment of panic disorder: the comparative efficacy of imipramine, alprazolam, and trazodone. J Clin Psychiatry 47:580–586, 1986

31. Modigh K, Westerberg P, Erikkson E: Superiority of clomipramine over imipramine in panic disorder: a placebo-controlled trial. J Clin Psychopharmacol 12:251–261, 1992

32. Mavissakalian MR, Perel JM: Imipramine dose-response relationship in panic disorder with agoraphobia. Arch Gen Psychiatry 46:127–131, 1989

33. Mavissakalian M, Perel JM: Clinical experiments on maintenance and discontinuation of imipramine therapy in panic disorder with agoraphobia. Arch Gen Psychiatry 49:318–323, 1992

34. Gardner DL, Cowdry RW: Positive effects of carbamazepine on behavioral dyscontrol in borderline personality disorder. Am J Psychiatry 143:519–522, 1986

35. Gardner DL, Cowdry RW: Alprazolam-induced dyscontrol in borderline personality disorder. Am J Psychiatry 142:98–100, 1985

36. Soloff PH, Cornelius J, George A, et al: Efficacy of phenelzine and haloperidol in borderline personality disorder. Arch Gen Psychiatry 50:377–385, 1993

37. Gardner DL, Cowdry RW: Pharmacotherapy of borderline personality disorder: a review. Psychopharmacol Bull 25:515–523, 1989

38. Elia J, Katz IR, Simpson GM: Teratogenicity of psychothera-peutic medications. Psychopharmacol Bull 23:531–586, 1987
39. Cohen LS, Heller VL: On the use of anticonvulsants for manic depression during pregnancy. Psychosomatics 31:462–464, 1990
40. Cohen LS, Heller VL, Rosenbaum JF: Treatment guidelines for psychotropic drug use in pregnancy. Psychosomatics 30:25–33, 1989
41. Rieder RO, Rosenthal D, Wender P, et al: The offspring of schizophrenics: fetal and neonatal deaths. Arch Gen Psychiatry 32:200–211, 1975
42. Nurnberg HG, Prudic J: Guidelines for treatment of psychosis during pregnancy. Hosp Community Psychiatry 35:67–71, 1984
43. Jacobson SJ, Jones K, Johnson K, et al: Prospective multi-centre study of pregnancy outcome after lithium exposure during first trimester. Lancet 339:530–533, 1992
44. Rosa FW: Spina bifida in infants of women treated with car-bamazepine during pregnancy. N Engl J Med 324:674–677, 1991
45. Ferrill MJ, Kehoe WA, Jacisin JJ: ECT during pregnancy: physiologic and pharmacologic considerations. Convulsive Therapy 8:186–200, 1992
46. Pastaszak A, Schick-Boschetto B, Zuber C, et al: Pregnancy outcome following first trimester exposure to fluoxetine (Pro-zac). JAMA 269:2246–2248, 1993
47. Calabrese JR, Golledge AD: Psychotropics during pregnancy and lactation: a review. Psychosomatics 26:413–426, 1985
48. Viggedal G, Hagberg BS, Laegreid L, et al: Mental develop-ment in late infancy after prenatal exposure to benzodi-azepines—a prospective study. J Child Psychol Psychiatry 34:295–305, 1993
49. Committee on Drugs, American Academy of Pediatrics: Trans-fer of drugs and other chemical into human milk. Pediatrics 84:924–936, 1989
50. American Psychiatric Association: Diagnostic and Statistical

Manual of Mental Disorders, 4th Edition. Washington, DC, American Psychiatric Association, 1994

51. Stone AB, Pearlstein TB, Brown WA: Fluoxetine in the treatment of late luteal phase dysphoric disorder. J Clin Psychiatry 52:290–293, 1991

52. Brantigan CV, Brantigan TA, Joseph H: Effect of beta blockade and beta stimulation on stage fright. Am J Med (suppl 3B):17–21, 1986

53. Liebowitz MR, Schneier FR, Hollander E, et al: Treatment of social phobia with drugs other than benzodiazepines. J Clin Psychiatry 52 (suppl):10–15, 1991

54. Leibowitz MR, Schneier F, Campeas R, et al: Phenelzine vs atenolol in social phobia: a placebo controlled comparison. Arch Gen Psychiatry 49:290–300, 1992

55. Fiore MC, Jorenby DE, Baker TB, et al: Tobacco dependence and the nicotine patch. JAMA 268:2687–2694, 1992

Index

Page numbers printed in **boldface** *type refer to tables or figures.*